DEFE
ADVENT
SCHIZOPHRENIA

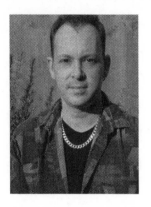

by Richard M Clements

'One million people commit suicide every year'
The World Health Organization

Dear Dinnen,

Staring through a thin camouflage of psychiatry, and the lens of a camera, all the events portrayed in this book are absolutely real and actually happened. I hope ~~that such truthful~~ information is everything you want it to be...

Richard x

Published by:
Chipmunkapublishing
PO Box 6872
Brentwood
Essex
CM13 1ZT
United Kingdom

http://www.chipmunkapublishing.com

Proof-read by Zahira Araguete

AUTHOR'S NOTICE

The multi-talented author, artist, and filmmaker Clive Barker is the innocent focus of my story. The memoir is entitled: "*Defender: adventures in Schizophrenia*," and portrays the extended reality crises of mental breakdowns. Outlandish and fantastical, this disorder often has a role model within a berserk and intricate background. The celebrated Mr Barker was the fulcrum of my own. I believed him to be the 'evil one' – the unknowing antagonist – in a reality that was dangerous only to myself. I could share it with no one else, and I could not choose or *voluntarily create* any part of this story.

"*Defender*" features a phantom telepathy with celebrities. Hearing 'voices' is a symptom of the illness but I was afflicted with other psychoses long before I first heard any of that horror. This is the whole story, written from my perspective. Within these pages there is *no connection* to common accepted reality. It isn't fiction yet reads as a memoir unique to myself that has no facts in it either – gun-less shootings, victimless murders, sunless dawns.

I would like to stress that *Defender* is entirely about mental illness and I'm *sorry to anyone,* particularly Mr Barker, who may be offended by his or her portrayal within it. While continuing my course of psychiatric drugs this book has been a cathartic self-therapy. By the time I began re-drafting it I was feeling very well. "*Defender: adventures in Schizophrenia*" may educate and entertain many people, but writing it also opened a door through which I have passed. In comparison to my apocalyptic beliefs of years gone by our sensual world is safe and my place within it is nothing as terrible as it had once seemed. Again, I apologise to anybody I have defamed in this writing but through it I am finding myself a whole person being made welcome, at last, in the Real World.

RICHARD x

This is a memoir from the battlefield of the psyche. It is a hazardous environment. The choices made there can be as pivotal as facing down a firearm in the Material Plane. You might think the gun to be far more lethal than the gibbering ghosts and wisps of its custodian's mind, yet blood is spilt in the killer's imagination long before his finger slips through the trigger guard. Mental afflictions can carry people to places equally bleak, yet their weapon of choice is almost always aimed at themselves. Suicidal courageousness, that impression of a final act of 'gallantry' is a *dire* illusion. Schizophrenia (psychotic episodes of self-harming, paranoia, perception, hallucinations, "voices", personality, and other disorders) affects 1% of us. That is over 10,000 sufferers living in London alone, and, like the landing craft pouring out young lads onto the bloody beach at Omaha, schizophrenia is up there at the Front and is still little understood.

Assuming a sick person volunteers for treatment at all finding suitable medication to aid recovery is experimental. It takes patience – hence a sufferer in a hospital is usually termed a "patient". When the right medication is prescribed it can save and alter lives yet even an accurate drug, if used for too long or at too high a dosage, can induce physical difficulties. Years ago three of my hospital friends were accidentally over-dosed with the 'common neuroleptic' drug *Haliperidol*. One young woman had to have her spleen removed. An elder woman is wracked still to this day by continuous muscular spasms. And Jason, who I met in 1990, was overpowered so badly he bit out his tongue. He was only sixteen at the time.

The worst and weirdest symptom of schizophrenia is the phantom 'telepathy' of voices. They exhibit independent personalities; can use accents previously unknown, express in languages you've never heard before, come obsessed with death, opinionated, often hallucinated, and swear rotten. They can accompany psychotic beliefs rarely discussed and they can talk to you even when you are asleep. And there may be no escape without help. My theory is that 'voices' are examples of broken consciousness induced by mental or cerebral damage, through such as drugs, mental abuse or head-injuries. They are shrapnel of the mind that poach independent neural nets of the brain and start talking. So the sufferer's mind becomes like a train running off down the track without anybody real in the driving seat while the psychiatrists try to safely de-rail it before it knocks anyone over. For myself, I've chosen to continue taking the new 'A Typical' anti-psychotic drug Closapine because it has

given me happiness beyond all expectations. I am thirty-four years old with brown eyes that are dark, and deep. I've been taking a small handful of these tablets for four years and it is working. I won't refuse it in the foreseeable future but it seems that in comparison to the time span of my conflict I've been well for a short time only.

Time and again sensitive and gentle, often creative, people are dragged down into places as close to Hell as any living person can languish in. Some psychiatric terms I've found degrading: 'liquid cosh', 'mental illness', 'pin-down', 'tribunal', 'catchment's area', and 'restraint room' – all is jargon that never helped anyone. Extreme over-dose is rare and the medicated path, though sometimes subject to side-affects that confusingly need to be dealt with by other, further medications, does promise a real chance at freedom. The unmedicated path is like a spiral stairway leading down to a dreadful yet perhaps familiar existence of demons and angels, alien conspiracies, love and hate. If the sufferer is blessed, or lucky, they may come back. It is possible to migrate beyond merely existing and throw away the crutches of defensive inventiveness. Be discharged from the microcosm of ward life into the macrocosm of the world and return to the sensual moments of life. And the longer stayed out of hospital the less chance there is of going back.

When this story launches into the telling of my experiences as though fact it will actually refer little to the effects of drug treatment because I secretly rejected most of it. I chucked out the pills, as many as I could, rebelling against involuntary treatment under Sections of the Mental Health Act *(1983)*. With the exceptions of being occasionally forced to take it and being reduced into a wreck of a man, I have 'palmed' hundreds of them. A pill in the hand is worth less than two in the bushes. I used to say: "Drugs got me into this mess and they won't get me out," I said but I didn't really believe that. The circumstances of my becoming a *Defender* of the Earth had been on the cards since we came down from the trees. It *always was* going to happen, an inevitability proved by a million thoughts, a thousand co-incidences. And when this 'latency' was realised, as a war the medium of telepathy became its own verifier. So I threw out the pills, not able to be understood, believed, or helped.

In this memoir I present truthful events as accurately as I can from the angle of a unique reality. It will be told from the history within, from the first person perspective of a victim becoming a warrior. A reader become familiar with this method might use logic to find poor continuity, gaps, and loopholes in the text but I wasn't a logical man. It begins as all of us do: as a child. Except that my childhood was damaged and terrible, and I didn't know it.

I had a privileged upbringing, lucky if you bare in mind the horrors of being a broadcaster of telepathy since being a toddler. I was raised on a muddy island called Mersea. The house where we grew up, my two sisters and I, is a mysterious place. There are exposed beams, paintings, and varnished wood. Dusty silver shines through diamond pane windows in the dining room. There are enigmatic ornaments and loose carpets under threat of occasional sparks from the lounge fireplace. Ivy climbs up outside but not Poison Ivy. It is a beautiful place indeed; yet, often, I didn't sleep well there.

My earliest memory is of being carried out into the garden on a warm summer night in 1969. I remember it from a divorced perspective, a glimpse of myself as an infant in the arms of my Godfather, Uncle Keith. He showed me the Moon and "moon" became my first word: not Mummy or Daddy but *"moon"*. The Enemy heard my childish thoughts and baby instincts (non-telepaths are known as "Naturals") and since one day I was to become the so-called 'Second Coming', I suffered years of cruel manipulations beneath the shadow of Anti-Christ figure Clive Barker.

He was brought up on his own Mersey, in the city of Liverpool sixteen years before me and he brought together a unit of some of the world's most terrible men. Manipulating thoughts, like altering an opinion is generally known as "pushed-sub-thought", or just "push-subs". A *"scu"* is the subtle-body a telepath can use for what Naturals call astral projection and Barker used his to alter me when I was little trying to prevent the man he feared I would become. This is a list compiled from events that took place while I was about four. I know that because my sister Ellie shared the room with me from the age of three and she was a baby in her crib next door when it all happened. It is a catalogue of vindictiveness based not only on the roots of deficiencies revealed later – such as the fact I couldn't read properly until I was about eight – but also from events I can actually remember: they altered visual perception, exacerbated ear/nose/and throat pains, inflamed cold sores (later); damaged my eyesight; caused Dyslexia, fear of darkness, a frightening belief in 'nullility' (non-existence) at death, odd flashes of self-doubt, hyper activity, nightmares, hyper-sensitive skin, fascination with fire, sleep damage, and other such psychological vandalism. It is a legacy so terrible it took over two decades to undo.

I awoke from sleep, once, and was terrified because I couldn't see a damned thing. I got out of bed with hands flailing as though blind. The room was utterly dark, as black as nothing. There wasn't even a sliver of light under the door and I stumbled about, increasingly frightened, until I found a path to my parents. 40% of my age group were afraid of sleeping without a light on and these days our children's generation are afraid of the dark also but the statistic has doubled to 80%. Maybe it's some kind of sensitivity to the Earth's difficulties, I don't know.

Two and a half decades later Barker admitted (telepathically, as always since I began to 'hear' in 1997) that he had been trying to show me, that night, what *nullility* was like, a word also known as *'not'* that means the ceasing to exist of the soul, and I've had some glimpses of such a destiny myself in this war but it is *his* fear. When I was four I began to wear eye spectacles, likely easing my fear of darkness and Dad gave me a night-light, a small ceramic mushroom with an orange bulb; sometimes yellow. It had little windows in it and a door, and if you looked through the windows you could see these little mushroom people. Nevertheless, there came the nightmares.

Many bad dreams, perhaps psychologically tailored for me by the Enemy that they visualised into my "imager", often sent me off often crying to my parents' door. In the earliest I can recall it was night and I was being chased down the road by a yellow sodium lamp on a post. It had a wig on it, coming after me, and it was making screeching noises. Mum tucked me back into bed and suggested that I dream of fields of strawberries. I tried to but I never did. For those active early mornings my parents used to leave a string of toys from my bedroom door, down the corridor, and down the stairs. I've been told that one winter night, when I was about three, my mother awoke with a feeling that something terrible was happening downstairs. She went down to the lounge and found me in there lighting candles. They were

burning everywhere, pretty lethal. Some had toppled over and all were threatening to burn the house down. She saved us.

Going upstairs in those days at night was scary. The steps were lit, the dining room unlit. There was an old grandfather clock in the deep end of that room that terrified me – bad magic in the darkness that, later on, scared my sister Ellie with the same terror. Barker called it a Balrog but the affects of magic, genuine Magic, only exists through the highest example of human evolution: *mind-to-mind communication.*

Unseen beyond the knowledge of Naturals, the *'mind life'* of a telepath might be seen (if known about) as being a lot of fun. Yet telepathy is another, complicated, secret life – which has, I hope and assume – kept the Earth safe from serious harm. Many have occasionally come across the practitioners of good or evil magic, known as white or black *"Rapturers"* and Barker is the master of the Black. The word 'Rapture' was probably plucked from the Book of Revelation, in the Bible, in which The Rapture was the essence of the final conflict between good and evil. In other 'vicinities', in other planes of existence (other Places – *not* other *dimensions*) they can move between dividing Veils and can sometimes attack with targeting gestures called *hand rapture*. But they mostly affect the material plane body with the act of Imagining upon it – imagination applied to physical senses which become solid, smelt; felt – and painful. I know this. I've been at the brunt of such attacks for decades.

Insecure children like myself, usually have a comfort toy and I had many, all of them similar: Soft pillow cases I used to call "pilly" which had originally carried the scent of my Mum and Dad's bed. A top corner of the soft cotton, changed about, was the part which I petted, called a "corny". Over twenty-five years ago I had a "pilly" on my bed illustrated with a cartoon dog called Fred Basset, asleep on one side and awake on the other. I didn't like Fred much initially. But I'm not afraid to admit now that he made a comeback to my bed a few years ago. 90% of the time it's on my bed even these days and – incredibly – my mother recently found another one such pillow case in a charity shop, which takes up the other 10% of bed space! If there are any pretty women out there reading this we could have 'his n' hers" Freds on our bed but my petting will naturally be heavier and concentrated on other places!

At nursery school I had once been painting. Like a baby Grand Master, I stood before a very short easel, most likely with powder paint on sugar-paper, and daubed a picture of home. It was a square house with a triangular roof and I painted Mum and Dad outside it. Since I don't remember my baby sister Ellie cuddled in the painting I must have been young – three – and when the teacher asked: "What is it?" I looked back at it and I couldn't see it anymore. During a brief alteration to an adult's perception it had become a mess. I've gathered since that Barker can't stand, never could, for me to achieve anything.

I mislaid my "pilly" a few times. One afternoon after I lost one I was looking around the house, dismayed, and I remember looking along the upstairs landing wailing: "pilly, pilly, where are you?" and then I suddenly felt as though I was some kind of infantile fool, faking it. I was shocked. Even before that apocryphal push-sub, I was with my parents on a walk along the fresh air of Coast Road once and suddenly felt that I was far too old to be in the process of being pushed about in a pushchair, yet most probably kept the thought to myself. I kept many thoughts to myself… festering. I had an old pony called Shane. I always felt like a baby idiot riding him and on a Saturday I was usually driven berserk to watch a Gerry Anderson sci-fi program called Space 1999 instead.

Magnified by my father's dreaded Old School Tie slipper punishments, for years and years all I wanted to do was something – anything – to make him proud of me. Yet learning was hard beneath Barker's fist and my school reports were always shit, and I started stealing. I took it as a boy wanting secret choc-ices, or chocolate from vending machines, was even driven to try to save it at the Post Office. This secret life made home-affairs seem contrived. I was entranced by the power of coin. My pocket money had been 50p to £1 a week, and one weekend I won a fruit-machine jackpot of £60 that likely had come from a force telepaths call 'Kaos'. The consciousness within chaos, called Kaos – Lord 'K' – of which there is a Black as well as a

White Lord, the white that can paint skies that are never twice the same – *singularities* – and which communicates through co-incidences called *synchronicity*: Lord 'K'... yet wherever it had come from that jackpot did me no good. It was a lot of money for anyone, let alone a boy of nine. A progressive sub-thought drive, by the Enemy, and I became a devious gambler for the next two decades, a thief and a liar.

When I was about six, at my first real school, I used to enjoy the feeling of my little palms pressed together in prayer. I was fascinated by the sacrifice of the Lord Jesus. Beyond the upper-school buildings on a path near the skirt of the farthest playing field there had been a broken fence that had leant against an old tree. I used to stand on that fence, with my back against the wood, stretching my hands to hold two outcroppings of twigs, re-enacting the Crucifixion. It felt right, holy. I occasionally spoke to other children if anyone walked passed but I was almost always alone there, and content.

As a little boy I had liked ducks, and oranges, but I was to realise it later. I knew it had been true because I would reflect on my parents giving me models of ducks on special occasions and wondered why. And Mum offered orange fruits regularly later in life and again I wondered why then understood it was because I had liked ducks and had eaten many oranges when I had been little. A lot of my childhood memories, happy moments, have been erased but some survived Barker's deletion.

Aged seven to eight years my Dad bought me a reflection of sailing, his own leisure interest. Mersea Island, which farms so-called 'Colchester Oysters', has a huge pontoon and so many colourful moorings it looks a bit like a balloon party after the Great Flood. It has been a focus of leisure boating and yacht racing for over a century. Dad gave me a sailing boat: a small fibreglass 'Optimist' class that was about the size of an average bathtub, with one sail, and it was bright yellow. I fixed bubbly letters down either side spelling her name: which was *"Barnacle"*. Ellie was given one also when she was old enough.

Summertime on the estuary, sitting in *Barnacle* wearing a big orange life-preserver, I hauled the mainsail 'sheet' with my left hand, the tiller in my right, cutting a clumsy but sure route between the buoys. I remember one hot day. The water was washing behind my rudder in a bubbling wake sparkling in the August sun, and I tasted true freedom, then... My father regularly encouraged me to try sailing on his larger boats but it was boring. It missed the point. In *Barnacle* I could push the rudder away from me – to sail left, or pull it towards me – to sail right, however the inclination took me. I answered to no one and guided my boat as freely as one of the gulls swooping and squawking in the sky overhead. One day, I would like to sail again in two small single-handers, island hopping from beaches of white sand and palm trees in crystal clear waters; a boat each with my lovely wife-to-be...

I loved stories too. Dad used to read *Winnie the Pooh* books to Ellie and I, and we probably got him to read *'Guinea Pig Podge'*, a slim book I remember lying about that had a picture of black-berries in it. We used to make up and act in plays, for our folks, writing out ten pence tickets. Aged five to six, unable to read myself yet, Dad got hold of two cassettes of the BBC Radiophonics Workshop's 1970s adaptation of a story by J.R.R. Tolkien. Cuddled up in a duvet under the lounge piano, cornicing pilly, I lay in a dark as mollifying as my mother's womb with imagination my light.

It had been The Hobbit, utterly beautiful, narrated by Mr Williamson alone – one man who gave a perfect performance of all the voices. The left speaker had been at my back, a Leek 'Sandwich Box' of quality; and the story had had lovely music and excellent sound effects. I had been exquisitely possessed. It was the happiest moment that I ever had as a child. When eleven, at my first boarding school in Felstead, Dunmow, Mr Andrews – the Headmaster – sometimes treated us to a tape story before sleeping. He had recorded a few frightening tales with his friends (like they had had their own Radiophonics posse) and one had been called "99 Bonk", an enjoyable spine-tingler about a giant centipede with a leg missing. One night I lent Mr Andrews the two Hobbit cassettes to play to the dormitory but the first broke and I have never heard that version since.

I hid my soft chequered "pilly" under my mattress, vital for getting off to sleep. A few friends in Felstead played war-games with me yet some boys in my Form cramped this outlet with sarcasm. Three times I found packets that somehow still contained cigarettes – and was *push-subbed* to make a big deal of not having smoked any when I handed them into the Headmaster. Our English teacher, Mr Fitzgerald, was a bumbling, intelligent and kind-hearted man. 'Fitz' used to allow us to play his LCD handheld games and in June and July he sometimes got us up at seven AM while others slept to go swimming. We crossed the grass to the outdoor pool, all essences all freshness, with bath towels rolled up in our arms. We dove through the cool surface that shattered into sparkles of light and I loved it underwater – that was how I had learned to swim in 1976/7 – and I fetched things off the bottom without my glasses, flipped about holding my breath. I pretended that I was a dolphin and told others, (maybe I even believed it), that I had been once, or come, somehow, from a dolphin.

At ten I read adventures like C.S Lewis's *'Narnia'* stories, and *Alfred Hitchcock and the Three Investigators*. In the excitement of a book I used to read after Lights Out under my covers. The Dyslexia, which had slowed me down for so long was cured by trips out of school to an old doctor called Mr Jolly. Dad drove to his house in the dark with sealed boxes of picnic stuff; sandwiches, an apple, a Penguin biscuit. I used to imagine the lights on the dashboard were those of a spaceship. Mr Jolly taught me to read and write based on phonetics. Not once did I get bored. These days if you were to look at the first draft of this book, pages that took a long time and a lot of magic to hand-write, you would see no such mistakes.

One afternoon the Headmaster's wife summoned me to see her. I stood before her, curious and worried. She was a blonde woman in her forties at the time with a foreign accent. In the Matron's office, with another woman present, she said: "This disgusting thing has been handed to me." I was horrified - *in her hand was "pilly"!* "It was found in your bed, grotty boy." Quaking, I found my voice. I asked her "What are you going to do?" and she replied, like a viper: *"It's a filthy rag and I'm going to burn it!"* I was utterly traumatised. I never grasped then, aged 12, that the real subject may have been an accusation of masturbation. I cursed the monstrous bitch and cursed myself for not arguing my side but I've always hated adrenaline. I have lost myself to rage only two or three times in my entire life.

It was fantastic when Dad picked me up in July after the last day of the summer term. We loaded my big aluminium trunk into the Rover, heavy with possessions, and I was driven home feeling joyful. Summer holidays were full of games and seemed long and sunny. In one game that Ellie and I called "Flies and Spiders", we dressed up in tough sailing jackets and climbed the inner branches of a big rhododendron. At the peak we jumped off in a floppy and probably dangerous fall back through the bush. I used to make summer cocktails: orange barley water in a tall glass with a straw, ice and a slice of real orange. We played 'kiss-chase', had water fights, and trips to Pick-Your-Own strawberries, and less dangerous games like "Socrates" in which we used to hit a ball of socks up onto the roof and back with badminton rackets. But as a boy I started to develop a huge appetite for something else – film.

Projections at junior school, on rare occasions, like *"The Italian Job"*, often found me in trouble when I would have to spend the entire movie facing the wall of the Headmaster's corridor. I slaked most of my desire for film during holidays. 'Star Wars', which I saw in a cinema in 1977, was the most amazing thing I had ever seen. Near the end, when the first

'X' Wing fighter dove into the trench of the Death Star, my stomach rolled in a physical wobble of sympathy for its pilot. One birthday I was taken to see a James Bond film, most probably a Sean Connery, a fatherly figure, and when I left the cinema I couldn't stop smiling for hours! Another great treat was to watch the BBC 1's slot called *Saturday Night at the Movies*. And when I was older, on weekends home, I was sometimes allowed to stay up very late and my favourite books and films joined the horror genre.

I hated baths and showers at Felstead and rarely brushed my teeth. I sometimes sat in classes doodling complex pictures of war: machine-guns and bombs, fighter-planes and artillery. I got the cane for being caught by Fitz "monkeying" around on a roof and Mr Andrews might have indicated to my parents that I was psychologically unsound. He once told them that all I had done during "the entire spring term was inventing an elastic-band gun". I started reading *The Pan Book of Horror Stories*, selected by Herbert Van Thal, and many of them were disgusting but I chewed through longer books as well, horror novels. The work of James Herbert (from which we read samples to the Matrons!) was banned.

I became obsessed with being "hanged by the neck until dead" and a shiver of interest used to sweep through me when seeing such an execution on a screen. A few times I threw a hangman's knot on a length of sailing rope over a tree branch – stood on a stool, 'feeling the weight' – most certainly because of a sub-thought-drive, until one day Mum opened her bedroom window and shouted down "what are you doing?!" Then I must have pulled myself out of the noose – and pulled myself together… for a while.

The Enemy made me feel sluggish in the mornings. On Sundays we had an extra hour's lie-in and that was satisfying. I've been asleep for over four years in the last decade and even now, with the date past the year 2003 and me past thirty years, older and uglier, the Sleep Raptures continue. They feel like a face flannel of corrosive acid wrapped around in the inside of my skull or a strip of metal pressed around the back of my brain. I believed for months that the chemical the body earned from good healing sleep was stolen every morning, before I awoke, even started to believe it was being sold! In June 1998 I recall leaping out of bed refreshed and happy at about 8am, but about decent sleep, that's mostly all I can remember.

Langley Park School in Norfolk was where I started smoking, during the spring term I turned from fourteen to fifteen. In those days I always had a healthy interest in psychic powers and arcane mystery and a few months shy of thirteen in Langley I wanted to try Astral Projection. With a set of instructions near my pillow, the lads and I went out one night to prepare for the experiment by exhausting ourselves.

The book said that an Astral Body can travel with a visual link through many physical as well as metaphysical planes (what I call *'vicinities'*) that it is connected by a kind of elastic silver thread which is connected to a Third Eye in the middle of the forehead. Egyptian sculpture often recognised this, exampled in the heavy gold death mask of Tutankhamun which has a riled up cobra snaking out of the mask's Third Eye. My friends and I, having climbed back up the rickety wooden fire escape, panting, got under the covers and tried the instructed method of relaxation and creative visualisation, to project. But none of us did. I personally found that at the stage of fully slack muscle, knowing somehow my body should become numb for it to work, I was thrown off the apple cart by salivation and swallowing. On other attempts, I usually fell asleep. But some people, telepath celebrities, *can* project, and much more besides.

This communication is possibly centralised in the bottom rear aspect of an evolved brain using a magical chemical called Thoracic Cortisone. The 'talk box', used initially, is abandoned in favour of easy-going communication with the whole brain later. A telepath's 'person' is constituted of six components: the *Vicinity one* / material body – a reservoir of *Phase Water* within that, which maybe called Spirit, a soul within that, which maybe called *a Feelie*. A *Fundament body* that exists in a vicinity called *The Circle of Fire* – that Barker said the soul travels *up* with-in – a *Control-Scu* in an interior vicinity of the material body that produces *Scu* and *Scu* that are connected, to begin with, through a silver thread to an Imager, to project to other telepaths so they can see through the other's eyesight. The subtle bodies of *Scu*, which allegedly have one eye (like a cross between Casper The Ghost and a Cyclops), can be trained, disconnected, and left for years on a kind of autopilot.

With an image-line on the *periphery* of centralized sight, selected by *Scu* trained in torture and combat, there is an almost subconscious *visual registry* they can move about called an "Attention Grab". They attracted my attention to things I wouldn't have noticed if I was alone. Sometimes I hallucinated little changes to the Grab, a "trick of the eye" that happened rarely but so fast it may have been a 'K' link. That part of my frontal lobe I'll call an Imager when it's hi-jacked for pictures by the Enemy, and as an *Imagination Drive* when I use it myself. My daily appetites – tea, coffee, cola – that most people couldn't live without for longer than a month (without going insane!), were also subject to manipulation. Such a need can become a physical ache generated by so-called "*Matter Collectors*".

One definition is the delivery of the desired matter, the fulfilment of a program (e.g. nicotine or caffeine) that is collected; and the other definition is like an unkind kind of exaggerated withdrawal symptom, an ache in the chest-area that becomes, itself, flesh painfully collected as matter, until it is eventually satisfied. A *Nussifier* is when a consumed thing is desired yet again because of itself – like cool seedless grapes popping with juices between the teeth, or dropping the salty stones of chewed green olives on to a plate – Mmm! Therefore a '*nussifier-matter-collector*' might generate a consumption causing more consumption. I was to discover that these mechanisms were mostly down to the hurtful act of *Scu* thrusting fingertips of their imagination into my physical body, with *pushed-sub*-thought. It left me being driven about in the past like Barker's pet robot. The manipulation was so continuous I had no instincts of my own and I couldn't have known the difference, but I had still never heard his name then, and I would not hear it until 1987.

When schizophrenia isn't busy being amazingly dangerous, it's busy being amazingly inventive. My psychiatrist since 1990 was an Indian woman with the presence of an elephant, who retired in 1999 and once, having learned for the first time a little of my story, exclaimed: "your psychosis is like a script for a Star Wars film!" It was one of the last things she ever said to me. Three years later, if I showed my current psychiatrist, a Chinese woman with the presence of a Triad accountant, the content of this story so far, in particular the narrative drive of the book as a believed reality, I would probably wind up Sectioned in hospital, again!

Langley Park was my last school, the place I sat for my 'O' Levels, like G.C.S.E but without the course-work. I got a new pair of steel rimmed glasses and chucked away those ugly brown plastic glasses of the N.H.S. They were exciting times. In spite of the dull daily life, ruled by bells, there was scope for rebellion. We explored the woodland growing at the back of the school and at night sometimes climbed about on lethal roof structures without safety harness or rope. Less dangerous and less healthy I was growing up into a world in which my raging hormones made my feet stink, a new world of masturbation and cigarettes; peeping and card-schools, and as few showers as I could get away with.

I enjoyed Art and pottery and I passed English Literature a year early with a 'C' grade. I played field hockey for the school 2nd XI team until the Enemy stopped it. During sport (allegedly since I had had my first smoke) they began to weigh down my muscles, exacerbate aches and pains, and strip oxygen out of my lungs with (a 'voodoo' or interior) "Air-Attack". Reeling with exhaustion while trying to play, I recall once wondering where this sudden weakness had come from... I had a sub-thought about cigarettes but it had been an insufficient explanation, didn't physically explain it, because I hadn't been smoking for very long. I remember thinking that. Even while running cross-country, years before, with Mr Andrews, I had found it difficult and rarely had more than *two* 'second winds' for six miles... Imagination. That was what I was about.

I performed in plays at Langley, or in the fiercely contested House Play Competition in which one year I won a cup for Best Actor. I wrote my first short film script when I was fourteen. Some friends of mine embraced the TSR role-playing game Dungeons & Dragons. When I first brought up the idea of starting a 'campaign' I was worried that they wouldn't get into it
– but they did – and I was The Dungeon Master! I designed maps on graph paper, used lead figures and gradually revealed the tunnels and rooms and corridors with Official snipped up mapping cards. Their adventuring was full of hidden traps, bloody fights, and occasionally I supplied the players' unexpressed needs – intoxicants, strange pets, gold, girlfriends – yes, they experienced the *romance* in D&D that they did not have outside of the game.

I watched as many films as I could, at Langley, mostly on weekend TV. At the beginning of a new term I was one of the keenest to sign up for the Junior Film Society. One winter we had the prospect of horror films. Fortnightly on a Friday night we skipped homework time after dinner, and piled into the lecture theatre to watch two wide-screen presentations. That winter the horrors were a B & W classic followed by a modern, colour feature. For example "*The*

Masque of the Red Death" staring Vincent Price, followed by "*The Shining*" staring Jack Nicholson, and I enjoyed those evenings. Although I liked the genre, one night I bit off more horror than I could possibly chew...*much* more.

It had been a Thursday, maybe, in about 1983. Certainly it wasn't broadcast on a weekend because we had to get special permission to watch it. To tune into BBC One, a film about the most unimaginable kind of war - nuclear war - called *"Threads"*, and it changed my life. I remember seeing the cover of the Radio Times. There had been a photograph on it that had excited me, of a man with a machine-gun wearing a Traffic Warden's hat and a gas mask.

I watched it and I learnt the true nature of horror. Set in Birmingham, the film showed the affects of fall-out from the days after the original war, showed the threads of humanity disintegrating as the film relentlessly portrayed the thirty years of nuclear winter that followed... my cotton self was gradually being stripped away, eating me to the core: I saw the unimaginable imagined and I was so traumatised by the terrible sickening hopelessness of it that when the film finally finished with a dire miscarriage I wept for a long, long time...

Soon the projection to others and the reception of charisma through emotional receptors across my rib cage became reversed. Barker applied what was later called a *Base-Controller*, made of *Dimension Two* (an evil material) placed between other people's senses and my chest. Not long after the pro-Earth lesson of *Threads* had been assimilated, what I had learned became unlearned. It became *REVERSED* also, into an attraction with dangerous people, a lack of patience with good people, a rejection of family, and an interest in the destiny of nuclear war that later was to develop into an obsession as unhealthy as my childhood fascination with the hangman's noose.

I read the novel of the movie "War Games", excited with its apocalyptic jargon like: Multiple Impact Re-entry Vehicles, I.C.B.M, DEFCON#, Projected Kill Ratios, Primary Targets; I found it chilling and the film enthralling. For the practical aspect of my 'O' level Computer Studies, I actually wrote a program in BASIC (on the BBC Model B, 32K computer) that visually simulated the military angle of the subject, the maps and missile paths, the intent behind the destruction. The cassette was sent to the Examining Board. I never saw it again.

My exam results arrived in the summer of 1985: Six 'O' levels at grade 'C' and a failure in Mathematics that I would have to re-sit. For further learning I decided to take Art, English, and Computer Science at 'A' Level. With a Red Marlboro habit of about 16 cigarettes a day, I returned to Langley to the world of Sixth Form education. We had the odd disco with girls from another school that rolled up our driveway in a coach that was like an alien spaceship.

We had the Senior Film Society, could take weekend leave to Norwich whenever we wanted and we each had our own single bedrooms away from the main buildings. The essence of this time was respect, maturity, responsibility, and serious learning – but it was in that aspect of serious learning that everything fell apart. I found 'A' Level course work to be more difficult than I had imagined it to be; less memorable and more complicated than any work I had tried before and it was ultimately so baffling I couldn't cope. So that winter term in the Sixth Form had been my last.

I left school in December 1985.

I remember my father saying to the others in the large hall of the Mersea Island Community Centre: "Richard's left school!" and it was *amazing*. The big question was what would I do next? The thought of a job, of a paid wage, was juicy. So I started working in the most obvious place – not requiring a C.V or an interview - on a construction site in Colchester being developed by my Dad and his colleague. The work was hard but the Enemy added to the aches and pains.

My legs and biceps were starved of oxygen and my daily application to the work felt like a sword fight in freeze frame. My developing muscles felt as though they were weighed down with bar bells. The weekly wage was £45 that I was putting most of aside for a camera called a Minolta 7000, the latest tech, and I actually thought I was putting myself into the work. But one afternoon a friend of Dad's got me up against the wall and told me I was a cunt about six times. I thought it was because I was considered a feeble worker that 'pulled rank' but with the beautiful Minolta under my belt and the building mostly completed, I gave up the job and I can't say I was sorry to see it go.

Dad convinced me to try education again, suggested a course in a subject that was a far cry from my creative interests, but I enrolled anyway. In September 1986 I started Business Studies. Again, under the *Scu,* getting up in the darkness at 6:45am for college all week then walking, breathe pluming out like freezing fog to catch a bus to Colchester, where I had to catch another coach to the seaside town of Clacton, then enter a class 'happy' at about 9:15am to learn a lot of boring shit... was it any surprise that *again* I lasted no longer than one term? If I had been a Natural (in another life, without telepathy broadcasting and a genuine interest) it's likely I would have not only have sustained the routine but I could have got the 'B' Tech National Diploma with a relative ease. But the word "if" is irrelevant, relative to Barker's intention to ruin the development of my 'Resume', my C.V, which had already started looking the worse for the crap and the lack.

That Spring I swooped back to Langley to re-take 'O' Level Mathematics but got sent off the property for insulting my old English teacher. I'm probably the only person who ever got expelled from a school he'd already left! Still never having heard the name Clive Barker before, at that stage I was still "unawakened". I might have been considered by other telepaths as a sleeping giant but I was really more like a hibernating squirrel.

In that February/March I applied for courses that were important to me. I was interested in the Lens Media and that summer I tried a different kind of lens: contact lenses. My will not to wear glasses overcame Barker's probable will to keep me in them. It was a little painful, a trial by fire, yet I did fold up my glasses within two weeks and I suddenly found someone in the mirror that actually looked quite handsome! Near this metamorphosis the postman delivered excellent news. I had been accepted onto a 'B' Tech National Diploma course in Audio/Visual Studies at a technical college 196 miles away, in Bristol. I found a bed-sit, made the financial arrangements, packed, was driven west by my father. I started the course in mid-September 1987.

As usual I had new paper and stationery that reflected a fresh attitude, a new beginning. My class was full of eighteen year-olds who were interesting, and I appreciated that they were interested in the audiovisual also. I had my Minolta with a long 70-210mm zoom and a 35-70mm, an allowance, and a dreadfully convenient credit card. I found an amusement arcade on the Gloucester Road for dipping into gambling. I began to make friends but I misrepresented myself. The city was rough. Re-moulding the silver spoon that I had been born with in my mouth into a bullet I contrived a past for myself that featured a "suspicion
I had killed someone accidentally in a riot". That had been *complete bullshit!*

There was a tall Welshman in college called Steve Preston, interested in Doctor Who, and he liked a blonde girl whose name I can't remember who I will call 'Shelly'. To be awkward I liked her myself. One of her associates was a big bloke, a bit of a comedian who promoted the 'wonderful affect of cannabis resin'. One evening 'big bloke' came round with some friends and it became the first time I had ever smoked the stuff. Shelly didn't believe how high I was protesting to be but then I threw up out of the kitchen window onto the front stoop two floors down. That might have verified my claim! Hash was another piece slotted into Barker's puzzle. But that autumn something took place as though attaching a baseboard to the puzzle, an event he could really build upon so that it (and I) could one day be framed and hanged. *I heard his name.*

In college in October, armed with a newspaper, Steve Preston told me of a new film release. It was an allegedly grotesque horror film called *"Hellraiser"* which had been written, produced, and directed by a man called Clive Barker. His was the most powerful name I had ever heard. It had an essence of a magical professionalism and a darkness that enraptured me, so we went to see the movie. I myself – often and as usual – was push-subbed to magnify the essence of my opinion. In the film demons called Cenobites passed through the Veil, creatures with blue skin and hideously bizarre body piercing. They came to punish the curious through a puzzle box with a bloody zest of flesh ripping hooks on flying chains. A kind of masochistic S&M hell, it was visually and psychologically revolting, and it pissed on many of my personal values. I had seen many horror movies in my time ('seen' I say because maybe 'enjoyed' isn't the right word) but I found *Hellraiser* to be truly memorable in its offensiveness, and swore – then – that I would never let a girlfriend of mine watch it.

Probably the oath wasn't particularly cared about during the revelations of later life, and a girlfriend in later life probably wouldn't have cared particularly about the revelations of the film, because *Hellraiser* only a problem in my perception. It was tailored horror, Barker's

chains to pull me towards his worlds. His hooks to pull me into a bookshop where his worlds awaited me. And, learning of a collection of short stories he had written called *'The Books of Blood'*, a bookshop was exactly where I went and when he netted me, the shelves from which the rest of his creative-paper-chase could begin.

I knew the city in which I lived, Bristol, was exciting, so I tried to play it safe. Yet I went to the arcade regularly and like any addictive institution it invited all the wrong people. I must have left Shelly to Steve because around that time I started seeing an art student named Vicky. I ate unhealthy food that I at least cooked myself, and kept fighting against the sleep rapture making it so hard to get out of bed. I still loved college but arriving there on time in the mornings was a battle I was beginning to lose. I had trouble with the process of making friends with people who were upright decent folk. It's possible that many of my associates thought I was a liar after that bullshit about riots; Shelly's mate 'big bloke' challenged me on the truth of it for certain. Yet the necessity to deny my gentle past with invention was down to the *Base Control Set*. Its reversal sparked making friends with good people unappetising and a fascination with danger. So, inevitably, one afternoon in the dubious 'safety' of the arcade I started talking to a charismatic foreign character off the street.

He was playing pool when I met him, a short yet powerful man. He was called Paul. He had been about 5'4", 21 years old, and olive skinned. I was draw into a few games and I began to assess him, or at least attempt to. From his street patois and his cheek about the police I gathered he was some sort of criminal. He strutted around the table swinging his two-piece cue of perfect wood like the antithesis of a majorette, his hands moving purposefully, applied to the game like those of a demon pianist. Maybe a car thief, so I thought.

His aura was paradoxical, an essence of electrifying poise yet with a terrible threat just beneath the calm. Paul had a gold loop glinting in his long black hair that framed his olive, aquiline, face, and a pencil thin moustache. He looked similar to Prince, the musical artist.
I learnt early that he was absolutely heterosexual. As with all bonding between straight males, women are mentioned first when the men first meet. Paul's most striking feature was his eyes, empty eyes, soulless, that betrayed nothing. He was a Greek Cypriot, working as a pizza chef in the family restaurant near the amusement arcade, and I admired him – a potentially violent man, yet nevertheless always in control. My 'respect' of him was about fear and the cat's curiosity of the *Base Controller*. It generated our friendship. I met him

several more times and Barker's next coup happened in November. I moved into Paul's flat looking for adventure.

We manually carried my things (for a long way, it seemed) up to his third floor flat in the Montpelier area of the city. We made an under-the-table deal. Paul would quietly continue to claim Housing Benefit and he would get my rent as well. I wasn't paying much, in fact the same amount as I had been paying for my old bed-sit, yet for a much larger room. My life went wrong quickly. I don't remember doing any home-work for the 'B' Tech and I was missing mornings in college because it was still so difficult getting out of bed – especially with Paul's small 'posse' thinking it was hilarious to come in late at night yelling "Richard, we're home!" Yet sometimes I exercised my fascination for danger and went out with them myself.

It had been partly late-teen rebellion, partly *pushed-sub-thought*, but also because I no longer had to contrive an exciting past. I didn't have to live risk through videos or lies. I had been a genuine lookout, a few times, in genuine danger. The life I had come to Bristol to lead had been that of a gentle and naïve student. Although I was supposed to be enjoying my studies, supposed to be learning my way to the keys of a fun job, it was all rusting before my very eyes. It was burning at the edges like my Diploma was on fire and had just seconds before it would be a crispy black thing dropped into a bucket, and I was burning it myself. I went along with some of their crazy plots and was too scared to confront Paul on any subject, was up to my neck in the bullshit of the lifestyle. Then finally I was lost to it. I had skipped twelve and a half days of college and I was kicked off the A / V course on 17th December, 1987.

Shortly after the 11am was expelled I went into the empty cafeteria and slipped 30p into the juke. Alone there I played two songs by Simple Minds: "Don't you forget about me" and "Alive and kicking". I sat and cried. I wept over a hopelessly ruined education, and in acceptance. I don't remember whether I prayed or not. For the third time I had lasted only one term in education. My noble purpose for being in Bristol was gone and I walked away from the college bidding it a regretful goodbye. I didn't think I could return home unless it was for Christmas only. There were mysteries brewing. My student life had been closed and a new life of many possible disasters had opened. I had no idea what to do next but I thought I would get the advice of a survivalist who really knew what was what. I would ask Paul.

Except for Vicky my pessimistic imagination didn't think any of my old college friends wanted to know me anymore. I felt that they saw me as a social leper representing their own fear of a similar fate. Young, and unemployed, I no longer had an umbrella to subconsciously hide from exposure to the very life-style that had put me into this terrible position. In spite of Paul's directions to sign on for Supplementary Benefit at the DHSS, I was learning about paranoia. It was a perception that called for both the escape into gambling and the escape into fiction. Barker's six novella collections called "The Books of Blood" were packed with outlandish stories, and all the front covers were illustrated with Barker's own bizarre paintings. I walked through the Broadmead shopping precinct late that December seeing many happy people buying presents for one another. There were children smiling, their parents bustling about with bulging bags to seasonal music, shop windows twinkling with lights. But I could have no part of it.

I remember reading no more than three books of Barker's stock prior to the New Year but what I did read was utterly weird, introduced by the theory that you can escape your hell by *tricking the responsibility* for your crime onto someone else. The stories won Barker the 1985 World Fantasy Award. The *Books* have a different air when considered as a collection; a different light, a different group atmosphere, its stories all gems. In retrospect I can look back on the majority of his work as being little more than targeting me for manipulation and the generation of *false telepath mythology*. But for those who read him for the first time I bet you can remember the almost primal interest his name awakened, remember the joy of wonders latent in his books.

As an outcaste, I left on the train from Temple Meads station and stepped off it in Colchester a few days before Christmas. I wasn't quite looking forward to the day itself. I travelled light with the subconscious fear that my father would invite me into the lounge and treat me like a naughty child. I had disappointed him again. I left my camera bag at the bottom of a wardrobe at the flat (after what had most likely been a *push-sub*) and after making sure Paul wasn't going to have any wild parties. The toilet had become blocked there. And my room was covered in stolen wheels, bicycles, busted stereos, tires, stains, and other garbage. My bed was comfortable but the most beautiful thing in the room, by far, was a big B&W poster of Kate Bush on the wall taken from the cover of her compilation album called *The Whole Story*. I had a wonder with her. She was a mystery, sexy, yet somehow motherly...

In a comparison of her essences, to the Anti-Christ's work, Kate's was enrapturing also but hers was the light of a White Witch, her art about something that I didn't understand then (and perhaps still don't) – the mystery of *woman.*

After stepping off the return train journey on 2nd January 1988 I let myself into the flat. The toilet was very bad. Since I had been away it had become a stinky blocked up quagmire of shit. I went into my room and found my camera kit had gone, stolen from the wardrobe, and my Katie poster had tears in it as though some bastards had been throwing pub darts at her. *Scu push-subs* found me thinking that Paul must have had a party after-all. They drove me down the road towards where he worked with a large kitchen knife in my jacket – but I came across him coming the other way. Walking in my direction he engendered in me that familiar fear. The *push-sub* intention to fight became the push-sub tension of flight and the confrontation had to be cancelled. We got talking. He had been making plans for us.

28

In January I accidentally flushed that toilet. A nightmarish gag had bubbled up and gushed all over the floors with a stench more terrible than the Aegean Stables and Barker's action must have been to 'take me out of the loop' because my memory is pretty good and I don't remember cleaning up that mess at all. I passed an evening's trial that Paul had arranged for me at the restaurant and then started a regular under-the-table job. I had an idea, twinkling, far away…we made ready to do a runner from the old flat. Paul's mother had invested her money into a trim three-bedroom house in Keys Avenue, in an area that was up the social ladder. Shortly afterwards I began to extend my idea: I was going to start writing, begin engineering my own destiny, plotting a horror novel of my own. We moved to the new house.

It was a tiny room but it was a compact, warm, in a pleasing little place, the stage where I began to eagerly soak up Barker's mystery. Laying comfortably on my duvet listening to an album by the band Tears for Fears, called *Songs From The Big Chair,* in particular some compelling extra tracks that perfectly reflected the essence of Barker's *Books of Blood* I was learning some right weird stuff. I was *push-subbed* to shoplift the books for an added spice, kind of like 'gifts from nowhere'. I took one off the shelf right out in front of a CCTV camera but I didn't get pulled up!

The stories felt 'epic', and I felt I was doing more than reading, that I was in fact digesting Secrets. Such as a journalist finding subliminal images in the art of a painter, who committed suicide, called *"Red for Chaos / Blue for Insanity"* in which the journalist obsessively paints the same scenes in the same locations until he finally commits suicide himself in the same way. This particular tale *had been* in the collection – that is a fact – but has been *withdrawn* from the latest editions since I read it. Perhaps that's because the mythology Barker created for telepaths had been the reverse of what he'd been teaching me. "Blue for Kaos" and "Red for insanity" just doesn't sound right after so long. So… had he been lying to me? *Or lying to everyone?*

These were afternoons with spring approaching, a promise of new growth and sunlight. The Enemy's first novel had been called *The Damnation Game* that needless to say was about gambling and for a change I might have actually paid for it! A riveting sink into the mind of gambler Marty Strauss, it was about both playing as well as watching, and about a mysterious card sharp who played for souls: and about paranoia, and about what price was worth being made a living dead slave.

Restaurant cooking was difficult but now my mind was sometimes away working for myself. I had mostly no common sense and almost no co-ordination and took a lot of stick for that from Paul, and from my two colleagues Nigel and John, but it wasn't all work, work, and work. On Saturday nights (while Paul was off doing the mysterious things Paul did) the rest of us took a couple of bottles of wine – which were like a bonus – with a video rental and maybe a 16th of hashish over to John's house where the three of us got ourselves basted like turkeys. But I was thinking about my future as well, thinking surely I had been born to do more than slave over a hot grill, and I knew inside writing was right. So in January I began to clank and 'ting' onto A4 pages with a tiny little blue typewriter.

Paul's T.D.C of a spidery moped (Police jargon meaning Taken and Driven Away) was stolen for my use. I arranged the 'ringers' (false number plates) myself, and it was great fun to scoot around on. Paul told me sometime he would ram-raid a photographic shop to replace my stolen Minolta. That never happened. I felt he was damaging my relationship with Vicky and there were some hurtful *sub-thoughts* about her illness, Bulimia. I don't know whether Paul had been ignoring my creativity or if he was curious but he never applied pressure to stop the work. Mostly his say about the noise of the typewriter wasn't serious.

My world became a comfortable routine: reading and writing, grill work and gambling. Paul took me to a casino twice and introduced me to a new dance music called Chicago *House*. Occasionally I wrote letters to my parents and for my birthday, in March, Dad bought me a brilliant little scooter. It was a cream 50cc Honda "Melody", ideally replacing the Puch, which had been ridden down the Avenue as far as the carburettors had allowed before it went spasmodic and broke down on a tank full of washing-up liquid, and piss.

Months passed. With the warmth of Spring Paul sometimes challenged me to fight him in the garden like we were a pair of jousting hares. There never seemed to be any apparent reason for this and I always backed down. I disliked hurting people and hated causing *others* bloody bruises. Paul told me that some of his homeboys had asked him why he condoned me hanging around the place. He may have answered it was a matter of *possibility*. He said he felt patriarchal towards me, like a father. He revealed that however much *he* was a destroyer, *I* was as much a creator and he wanted to have a character in my novel. Sometimes we worked on it together, when I sought his advice on street honour, theft, models of cars, and driving skills. Paul said that there was a high chance he would be going to prison soon. So I began planning the last chapter of the book.

It had been a Friday night in the house in the early summer of 1988. John, Nigel, Paul, and myself were all there. We had a mug of tea... maybe some alcohol. I left my wallet on the kitchen counter. It had a GIRO cheque in it, Housing Benefits money, and a full week's wages in cash. The wallet had gone and one of my three most trusted friends in the city had stolen it. I walked to Nigel and John's, challenged them to no avail. Walking back to the house on Keys Avenue Paul took me from behind the door, suddenly jumped me into a headlock. He knew about my accusations and challenged me to challenge him. He may have actually *been the one* who had taken it, but a *push-sub* of that so familiar terror later and I was lost. Everything was lost.

I'd been gambling up to my neck in water starting to boil. I was hopelessly out of cash and had a VISA card on the maximum £250 limit. With the theft of my wallet I couldn't afford to pay the rent and I wanted to go home anyway. I couldn't live this life any longer, so I told Vicky it was finished, done with... done with grilling, done with Paul, and done with the City of Bristol which is like a huge soft poisonous fruit. In the final chapter of my horror book Paul's part was to meet his death behind the wheel of a car.

In the book of my own story the first chapter of a young child's life grown into a young adult is now also at an end. Unlike Paul's character, I had survived. I had learned much about Barker consciously in those ten months, and been affected much by him much unconsciously during those months. Many others would follow. His army and himself had exerted masses of control... I had worked as hard as Barker wanted me to work... rested as long as Barker had wanted to me to rest... and played as hard as Barker wanted me to play. And although I knew nothing about this I had nevertheless matured and had no criminal record. Paul was going to prison. I had my health and I was alive and, that night, I telephoned home. I packed my things and Dad picked me up and drove me back to Mersea the next day.

CHAPTER TWO: *1988 - 1989*

When I got back to Mersea in August I had a different opinion of my own status. I had come from being a little fish in a big pond to being a big fish in a little pond. I was a hard man in a harmless place yet I had been away for too long. I felt tough, I went about talking "street", but I didn't know many people and I had to forge new relationships. As a user of hashish I was part of a social sub-group that meant making friends wasn't going to be difficult. Within a day of my return an old mate named Robert rang up suggesting we backpack it down to the south of France and it was a fine idea. Empowered with my parents' money I bought a rucksack and Rob's dad dropped us off in Dover. Our first purchase on that drizzly day in France was a beer each. It cost us much and we became worried about how long our money would last. We had only been in Calais for an hour! Robert and I shouldered our loads, hit the road, and it took us a week to hitch hike south.

Near the coast we caught a ride in a battered Citron 2CV. It was our second lift in such a car. As we were loading our packs into it a glossy red sports car pulled up behind us. There were three girls in it, gesturing, calling to us in French, and they were only wearing bikinis! After what had most likely been a *push-sub* of cowardly paranoia I rejected their offer because they might have been teasing us. If we turned down that certain ride in the 2CV those racy women might have had a great laugh, leaving us stuck there and spinning off in a cloud of smoking rubber. The possibility of "sleeping in silk sheets that night", as Robert had deftly put it, went with them.

Finally we settled in a seaside town between Nice and Cannes called Juan le Pin. We rested on the beach in darkness but for the moon. Robert was tucked up in his sleeping bag and I lay under a duvet with my head resting on a soft familiar pillow. We drifted off to sleep to the sounds of palm trees waving in the warm breeze and to the washing surf – were to sleep there, it turned out, every night because the official camping sites were too expensive. The entire seafront was composed of public divided with pay-as-you-use (peage) beaches. Sleeping on a peage we were awoken at about half past six every morning to the noisy up-roar of a beach cleaner that had been about the size of a combine harvester. I never did see it coming properly because I never had my contact lenses in at the time but it had seemed to me that this monster was not going to stop, that if you didn't get out of its path quick there wouldn't be much of a body left for the funeral and no one would want to use the beach for a long time.

Again, I was to change psychologically on that holiday, particularly in the aspect of my religion. Scantily clad women sun-worshipping on the hot sand drove my nineteen year-old hormones crazy. Deciding to address my lack of confidence head-on with a quick fix I visited a Private Shop in Cannes. I bought a sexy colour picture book staring teenage girls (who may have been over twenty, if you follow me) and returned happily with it to Juan le Pin.

Robert was becoming stressed about our beach-bum life, perhaps seeing more than he wanted to. I had lied to him a couple of times about weapons to spice up the adventure but much of what really bothered him was very real. One morning we were sitting with a few strangers outside a café having breakfast and during our espresso and croissant this car pulled up - and a man leant halfway out of a back seat waving a shotgun. Yet it wasn't an armed robbery. He was just boasting about it, pumped a round into the breech, saying (the French equivalent) of "Look at my new shot-gun!" and then they drove away. Robert looked stunned about this, his coffee cup perhaps suspended halfway between the tabletop and his lips. Nobody wants to see the dirt under the gloss on holiday but we had no campsite or B&B or hotel room to return to when darkness fell, just an assumption of safety. Rats scuttled amongst the detritus a few sections up from where we slept.

One morning a rat of the human variety struck. I'd been having a wash after we avoided being minced up by the monster beach cleaner, and when I got back I found my pack had been stolen. Going to report the theft at Antibes Police Station was Robert's final straw. With the report made, exaggerated with a dribbly anticipation of travel insurance, Robert arranged to go home. For myself I had been enjoying watching the young French people cuddling on the beach, or holding each other while strolling along the promenade, and I thought France was the most romantic place I had ever seen. Even without my pack I intended to stay. I remember standing on the train platform with the automatic doors closing between us. Standing in a 'T' shirt and shorts, with flip-flops on my feet and a towel in my arms, I weakly waved goodbye. Without a great amount of money or even a phrase book, Robert left me behind. The train took him.

With cash become a problem my parents wired more than I needed to a couple of their friends who were working on a motor yacht in Antibes Marina. I picked up the money and got a room in Juan le Pin. Soon I returned to the porno shop in Cannes and amongst the decor of magazines, toys and videos I recognized the words "jeune fille" on a couple of books, bought them, and opened up one behind a locked door in a café toilet. It was black and white and terrible. It had pictures in it of sexual bankruptcy, of insane photographs (like adults romping around in nappies) that had shocked me to the very core. I dumped all the books under a bush. Dirty inside, I walked down to the sea front where I could cleanse myself... and there before me was the deep blue Mediterranean ocean.

I buried my wallet under some of the smooth grey slates and marked the spot with a towel. Before God I began to swim from the water's edge along a line of yellow markers arrayed at 90 degrees to the beach. I swam from one to the next, needing a kind of baptism. Tired, I hung on to the last buoy and looked back at the coastline. It was a long 200 meters away, looking like a pretty panoramic postcard. I had become unsullied. When towelling myself down I knew it was done and I left France a few days later. As a Christian Soldier I slipped through British Customs carrying three knives I'd purchased in Cannes: a 3" stiletto and two identical 4" switchblades to defend the innocent. Whether I could actually cut anybody with them or not will never be known. I doubt it. I got through the (Nothing-To-Declare) area without incident. Back in Mersea at church on Sunday mornings I used to hide my studded belt and weapons under an evergreen bush. But there wasn't much soldiering to be done on a muddy island that is only six miles long. Gradually, I slipped away from church going.

Making new friends these days and fording that sense of separation that we build around ourselves, is difficult. Take London for example: ten million strangers that never talk to one another, who crush together on public transport fearful of sharing even a glance, wobbling along the Tube as far away from one another as three or four inches allows. Most friendships are cemented in sub-groups of modern life, such as snooker halls, gym clubs and adult education groups. Students use societies, white-collar workers have their wine bars, but perhaps the biggest and most all wide-ranging sub-group in society are the users of drugs.

It is a 'scene' that comprises of a huge scattering of individuals who spend so much time on the fringes of perception most are paranoid regarding anyone who doesn't do it. If you roll a joint at a party you share a common ground with anyone else that smokes it in the room. Become an "Us and Them" situation, total strangers can become instant friends. I made a bond with three men who were each from different backgrounds: a fisherman named Jason, a London merchant banker named Migs, and a guy who may have been a fisherman also, or a student or a fish processor or something, called Patrick. We were all linked through using resin. It has less to do with addictive qualities (marijuana and L.S.D. are not physically addictive) in my definition it is more a connection with law. I say a drug is either *illegal* or *proscribed* and extensive use can strand its users in a mental hospital at the last station on the railway of experimentation where all trains terminate.

That September my dad got back from seeing his stepfather in Majorca. He had bought a novel from a bookstall in the Departures lounge, read it, and, on getting home, had left it lying about. I found it on the kitchen table. It was a heavy paperback with a cover picture of a man glowing with light leaving footsteps in the snow. It was entitled *"Weaveworld"* and it was written by Clive Barker.

In this book I first read of *Rapturers*, in a novel that featured a fabulous world woven into a carpet. Within the story was the echo of the Barker's own fear of 'nullility', a monster of emptiness in the plot that he, himself, might have considered cathartic writing. A character trying to track the carpet down - named Shadwell – was a salesman whose jacket had a scintillating lining which offered whatever the mark most deeply desired, but were things that always fell to dust. Also in the plot were examples of sub-groups that were coined "Weavers" and "Cuckoos" – and I learned of a new expression that a push made me sit up and take notice. *"Look Between," said Romo. "Between what?" asked Cal. "Simply Between," he replied, as though the sense in this was self-evident.* But I wasn't to learn what that actually meant for another seventeen months.

That winter, in 1988, I was in the Spar shop in Yorick Road, on the island. I had been buying Marlboro and chocolate, or something equally healthy, when I found myself sifting through a small bookstand and I didn't need look for long. As I was reaching out to pick up a paperback entitled *"Cabal"* (which had a demonic skull embossed on a sunset, above a distant city on fire, on its cover) it became less of an *alas Yorick* and more of an *"Alas poor Richard I knew him well!"*, because Cabal is another Clive Barker novel. It is a riveting, 'tailored', work, which may have marked the true beginning of my learning curve.

Cabal features the unusual concept of the monsters being the good guys and the *bad* guys being the humans; of subgroups again, of "Naturals" and "Nightbreed". I believe synopsise of Barker's work are pertinent to my memoir, and *Cabal* has a particularly enticing plot. The protagonists in it Aaron Boone and his blue eyed raven haired girl-friend Lori. That Boone is on psychiatric drugs is written within three paragraphs of the first page. His psychiatrist is called Decker, who frames Boone for *his own* murders, which Boone believes he has done when he sees a sheaf of photographic evidence spilled over his doctor's desk. Decker tells him to give himself up, gives him a pill to calm him. The pill turns out to be a lab-quality hallucinogen. Boone is almost knocked down by a truck and in hospital he meets a stranger who is muttering about a secret home of monsters, a mythical place. "They forgive you there," Boone says wistfully to his new friend Narciss. And he goes off to find it. The city has a name with the essence of the word *Between*, which is hidden under a cemetery, and it is called *Midian*.

A proud creature with hair like dreadlock-snakes called Peloquin bites him that first night. Mere minutes later, Boone is shot to death outside Midian's gates by the police corps. He reanimates in the mortuary: become a living dead man because of Peloquin's bite. He can do most of what a Natural can do – think, make love (what else is there?) – but his heart is still and he has a strange new appetite for blood. He has become a monster, and seeks out his kind in the only place he can - under the graveyard with the Tribes of The Moon.

The *Nightbreed* welcome him, subject to Laws like *"What's below remains below"* and their own prophesy is that a dead man would save Midian from the Naturals. Lori tracks him there, darting between the monuments above ground pursued by the knives and button mask of Boone's insane psychiatrist. Boone breaks away and goes up and saves his loved one. Decker escapes. The enraged Naturals, led by fascist police captain Eigerman, city inspector Joyce, an apocalyptic priest named Ashbury (who himself becomes a monster) and Decker himself, come crashing down upon Midian, a lynch mob with guns. Boone had broken the Law. He broke it because of his love for Lori and because of him Midian is destroyed. It is an awesome and mind-bending concept.

In a first edition *Cabal* there is an author photograph and an illustration on the title page that are darkly inspiring. The title page features an 'ink press' of twin aristocratic creatures, linked by upraised hands, about a reflection of an equal pairing that is not referred to in any other way later in the text. The author photo itself awoke a jealous fascination within me. It speaks of an inaccessible arcane knowledge, Barker staring blackly into the lens with two or three small demon imps whispering secrets at his right shoulder and secrets into his left ear. And this artist's face, challenging his readers through this picture, was *almost my face.* I looked into mirrors in those days with wonder. I appeared like a younger version of Mr Barker (both our bone structures and hairstyle alarmingly similar), and with this blatant B&W evidence our blooming psychotic connection developed further.

That autumn I broke the ice of my own writing, kick-started a horror novel using a divided up short story on a Canon "Star Writer" with WANTED DEAD OR ALIVE written on the *Cabal* photograph that I had stuck to the wall. My book's theme was street crime, magic, and demons. The plot was entirely in my head, never annotated, and there is much in it that is autobiographical. I am going to re-write it in 2004, a good deed. Bad habits can be reconciled with actions like that. The root problem doesn't seem so bad when it's balanced. For an example we had a physics teacher called Mr Becket who had a heavy cigarette habit – he sometimes dipped out of classes – and he resolved this by (I once saw it with my own eyes) jogging around the running track while *smoking* at the same time! In my own case odd moments of paranoid guilt from using hashish with the lads was lessened knowing

I was a writer with a good novel in progress. And thoughts of my girlfriend Maria made losses at gambling seem almost unimportant.

Be it bad for some or good for some, a *Learning Curve* to me is a sequence of inner experiences that leads to a definitive conclusion. Other art forms were inspiring my progress, aspects in a life of discovery. The first three brilliant albums by the band *'The The'* led by singer/song writer Mathew Johnson, are in point: "Infected" / "Soul-mining / "Mind bomb..." Even *the titles* of the albums fit the pattern of a complete learning curve! The distinctive video of "Infected" is rated cert.18 because it is so psychological. I've wept over the second track at least twice. It is a song about a man who feels the need to prove to himself that he is still a man. He drives to an easy woman but when he embraces her part of him is watching the scene from the doorway singing, "I was trying so hard to *please* myself I was turning into somebody else" watching his body flop impotently in her arms singing, "I was trying so hard to *be myself* I was turning into someone else."

A lot of people past middle-age talk of 'about twenty years ago' as though it is a kind of mythical Golden Age when the days were sunny and care-free with less crime and more opportunities. It isn't true. There is always crime and life is almost always hard - even if it wasn't particularly hard for me - in Victorian times there were "Press-gangs", organised crime in the twenties and thirties, Teddy boys mugging people in the fifties, Mods fighting Rockers in the sixties and seventies, Punkish anarchy in the eighties, and desperate Crack Heads in the nineties. I've talked to patients in hospital before on the issue of their recovery. Many say they want to go back "to how they were 'Then'" before they were ill and this is another kind of mythical age. The past should teach us the present but is, nevertheless, past, and the more a person lives trying to be how they used to be the more they will change into a completely different person. I've told them so, learnt from *The The*. What's wrong with being a new person anyway? You won't make the same mistakes - you'll just make new ones!

I suffered a backache for over twelve years, an attack usually located in the same vertebrae about 3/5th s of the way up my spinal column. It hurt at home on a Sunday while we ate a traditional meal. I didn't rush my food because I was hungry I rushed it because of how painful it was to sit up straight. I was to learn later that it was some kind of drip device, a spinal tap to leech inter-dimensional spirit, the spirit of dreams – literally of *dreams* – called Quiddity. I have a stoop these days most likely because of that tap. It has made my 5'11" more like 5'9" and bad posture is something that I may have to address later in life. At least the pain has faded. They lost grip.

So, I wrote with my machine at odd times of the day and night, and I smoked hashish at the weekends. Dad said if writing was indeed my 'job' then I ought to get up at a decent time – and write 9 to 5. I had been getting out of bed near lunchtimes. I argued that the creative impulse couldn't be switched on and off at will yet, paradoxically, I've heard of authors talk about writing as a discipline to be done with regularity. These days I have found this possible and valuable. Dad and I fought verbally a lot and the months passed. I found myself working in the middle of the night but at least I was getting it done, and it was good. I wrote at a table in the same room I slept in, something I haven't done quite so much on this book. In the spring of 1989 Dad and I were still arguing. He said I was pushing a wedge between himself and his wife, my mother. But then, I think, he might actually have started to enjoy my writing, making the work and *our lives* so much easier.

The new dance scene of laser-guided "acid house" parties, fuelled by L.S.D, became known as the Second Summer of Love. My three friends and I were becoming intrigued with hallucinatory drugs because we were finding hashish delivered a blunt edge. We needed something new. L.S.D tabs, with names like 'bats', strawberries', 'jokers', 'microdots', usually generate only one extraordinary 'trip', one intensely beautiful glance into another world. Forever after that you can do as much further experimentation as you want with the stuff, fry your brain with it again and again, but I believed then you'll never return to that place. The cost of a tiny square of blotter acid in the autumn of 1989 (the *financial cost*) was £5. Although that's a hefty price by today's standards, for what it offered, an intense experience, opened a market to people who may have been too young. The drug was within a young person's price range and too cheap for the damage it can wrought on a tender mind. I had been twenty years old then and maybe tender myself, had I just known it, but when you are a happy adventurer it seems you can take on the entire world at poker and win every hand without a moment's bluffing! One night in the flat we took 2 ½ allegedly 'double-dipped' tabs each – and that trip had been really special; vinyl 12"s; strobe lighting, Pink Floyd... the next morning, about 13 hours later, we went into Colchester on a bus and we were still slightly high.

Tripping in both senses of the word, the top deck of our bus felt like a swaying helicopter flying under radar, and under the radar of the sober passengers sitting behind us. We walked through a peculiar town in which at one moment it seemed everyone we passed had been speaking a foreign language. In the central precinct I witnessed a strange place where everything seemed to be fake. The buildings were like cardboard: the bright shops windows like sugar-glass, the money changing hands like waste paper. Only one thing was certain. At the time with this heightened consciousness I could see into people, and their souls were looking out of their eyes!

I clutched at the wall of a shop where Jason had gone into to buy some boots and stood outside it like a man drowning in a seemingly ceaseless flow of humanity. I could see their souls, their bodies as machines, with masks of faces. Some of the babies in pushchairs seemed to have deeper eyes, older souls, than their parents. For me, this was an experience that verified re-incarnation as a working metaphysical system. The higher state of consciousness the L.S.D had produced had been inspiring: it had made fact out of nonsense! It had been an epiphany, (perhaps with Barker's manipulation), on my learning curve and if I had been interested enough to look at Jason's boots they probably would have looked a little fake also.

In the late summer of 1989, I was in a Dillons bookshop in Colchester when I came across a heavy novel called *The Great and Secret Show*. I picked it up immediately. It was also entitled *"The 1st Book of the Art"* and this had been Barker's latest novel, and I was very excited. Within its inner covers there are pictures of masks with blank, white, eyes - faces of the way people see themselves yet without souls looking through them. I knew that this large book had many *secrets within* and inside the prologue page is written an arcane statement that would evolve into the heaviest of Barker's unique myth:

"Memory, Prophesy, and Fantasy:
The past, the future, and the Dreaming Moment,
Between, are all one country, living one immortal day.
To know that is Wisdom.
To use it is *The Art*..."

The Enemy were shepherding me towards something huge. I would be too frightened to be awake within four months but there was seven years still to pass before I could hear them and engage them to war as a full 'receiver'. The fight was the third conflict, and it was to be fought in the mind. The Enemy's training of attack *scu* placed within my inner vicinity, and because of the long years of manipulation – which had been a kind of retroactive smear campaign – Barker perhaps avoided direct assaults upon me. Most of his own fighting had already been done earlier so, with progressive logic, he probably carried on as though it was business as usual: writing, painting, producing – I didn't realise. In the Bible is written that 'the end of the world will come like a thief in the night' and on the rear dust jacket of *The First Book of the Art* was a statement revealed to me, by a friend, that was to become reversed deliciously by the *Base Control Set*: ARMAGEDDON BEGINS QUIETLY.

CHAPTER THREE: *January – March 1990*

When the new decade began I resolved not to take L.S.D again. I had witnessed the reality it concealed and had learnt the secrets it can teach travellers in consciousness. There was no more digging to be done except for striking sparks into the unyielding bedrock of embryonic insanity. There was no more to learn. I was done with it but I passed through New Year with a slim book in my hands that was potentially more psychologically damaging than that wrought by the acid. Barker had made a film out of *Cabal* entitled *"Nightbreed"*. The book in question is called the *Nightbreed Chronicles* and it would quickly become more important to me than "*The First Book of the Art*".

Reflective forces are pitched together in that larger novel. A drug-using scientist called Fletcher, a kind man who had just "wanted to be sky" is hurled against Randolph Jaffe that became the evil force known simply as The Jaff (like *Jaffa* oranges). They had evolved through exposure to their invention (the 'Nuncio') and had become spirits. Fighting across the length and breadth of North America in an undetectable conflict both were so balanced neither could win. The Jaff's goal was to tear open a hole in reality using a power called *The Art,* to let the Dream Sea into the world, the spirit of heaven, called *Quiddity*, protected by a group called The Shoal. So the mythology goes, human souls swim in Quiddity three times: at birth, at death, and when you sleep with the love of your life for the first time.

The warrior spirits were driven underground in a state of weakness, into caves beneath the woods near the town of Palomo Grove. Hard rains, their place was flooded and some teenaged girls went swimming there. The Jaff went up through the water and laid a seed that would drive the women to get pregnant wherever men were available. Fletcher did the same. He had to match the Jaff. They wanted to continue their war through their children… but, years later, two of their kids meet in Palomo Grove and fall in love at first sight! Fletcher and the Jaff rise from the depths. They battle in the streets, Quiddity is opened by the Jaff's left hand and across the spirit sea is a force called the *Iad Oroboros* that want to gain entrance to and destroy our world. Yet another awe-inspiring plot!

The *Nightbreed Chronicles* contains over 40 photographs of monsters from the movie that all have extraordinary make-up. There's a paragraph written about the background of each by Barker himself. I found myself needing to call them *people* rather than *monsters* because to me they had all looked like unique individuals. These are the victims of the tale, staring passionately from the pages of Murray Close's photographs. There is a character called Vasty Moses, (the Moses of 'Corpulence', who would have wished to bring his tribe to true freedom if he hadn't been the last of them) and there is a photograph of Barker seated in front of Peloquin, the creature in the movie whose bite had transformed Boone into that attractive monstrosity. The Qualm creature stands proudly behind his director with an arm draped easily across his shoulder, and they look on with a hint of amusement and the confidence of unimaginable weaponry ready to deploy after the temporary cease-fire of their portrait. It is a challenging depiction of their alliance.

Then I set my eyes on the photos of Boone and Lori, the seeds of a learning curve that would sweep up everything and mark the beginning of what was to follow. I looked at the imagination of the filmmakers made flesh, adjusting my increasingly bizarre personal reality because of Lori's beauty, and because of her lover frozen in his bestial state, a growling monster with teeth strong and pointed. I wanted these consequences in the Material Plane, both. My need for a persona, a lover, and a future, was fuelled by the tract written about Boone as being: "The 7th Saviour, a trampler and a transformer, a scapegoat and a monster… a Hero for the Night."

In the photograph Boone is to be viewed expressing rage I had almost never experienced before. Obviously pictured at some point *after* he had received the bite that had terminated his psychiatric diagnosis, his illness of 'un-belonging' had been declassified when he found his way to Midian, his true home, which sharpened the knives of his murderously insane psychiatrist, Doctor Decker (played by a soft spoken Canadian horror director David Cronenberg). To Midian, then: "The city where all sins are forgiven" where he found the stonework and earth of a real place, proved not to be a figment of a psychotic's imagination after-all, yet for him a fact – as were the creatures beneath it.

When I got back from a holiday in mid February 1990 I was soon to begin identifying these 'monsters' as metaphorical of my own family. I also believed that other creatures within the *Nightbreed Chronicles,* depending on the attitude and actions of my current 'self', were alternative personas other than Boone for an identity. It was one delusion of many without doubt exacerbated by regularly smoking hashish with a new friend I'd met at the flat named Tony. In the darkness of the countryside, as though his Ford Granada was a submarine in which we talked, we grew wiser. Listening to the haunting album *"Zoo Look"* by Jean Michel Jarre our learning curves merged and I quoted a couple of songs to emphasize my opinion, such as from the album *Mind Bomb* released in 1990, a track by 'The The' called *Gravitate To Me* with the lyrics "you're like a boat without a mast, struggling with the tide of destiny between the future and the past." The lovely Kate Bush released her album "The Sensual World", also in 1990. The track called *Love and Anger* has the lyric "We're waiting for the moment that'll never happen, living in the gap between past and future." I wondered if L.S.D perhaps allowed a glimpse into this 'dreaming moment'. A terror of the drug is the question as to whether you'll never ever 'come down'. If any of you readers out there are acid 'space-cadets' let me ask what *you* would do if you stayed living in that madness for life? In my own example the concept of a 'flash back' later was something I dismissed as impossible. Yet these days, even over a decade later, I sometimes to an extent still see unexpected shapes in a continuously and very slightly rippling *now*.

Without addressing the issue in our first conversations – it was a taboo subject – it was becoming clear to me that Tony and I were at war with paranoia, that our goal was to be released, freed from it. Feeling a new sense of freedom I deployed my strength on a trip to London. I an application form for the London International Film School in my bedroom that I had never posted because of the examples of fruitless education on my shitty resume. One day I overcame my awe of the place, and said "what the hell!" so on a Wednesday, when the school was open to visitors, I went up there on the train. In Covent Garden I found it beside a dance studio and had a lovely time looking around it.

In the cafeteria there I met a young American man who told me he was travelling around himself to find the best course in film. My naivety, my complete lack of any real knowledge, was revealed when he asked after my favourite director. Approximately, I had replied "Kurt Russel, maker of *Lair of the White Worm*" and the man said he'd never heard of that particular director. What I had actually meant to say was *Ken* Russel and although later, when I had realised my slip, I figured the American had been nasty, it is perhaps proof the entertainment industry breeds such an attitude in some people because it is the most terrifyingly competitive of all professions.

I walked out of the school into the sunshine and saw some trendy brooches for sale on the other side of the street. I crossed the road with a flare of interest. Pinned to the board were about 60 badges; fashionable pop merchandise, occult badges, (fashionably occult badges) football clubs, makes of cars and bikes. I wanted to buy one that expressed my feelings about L.S.D but encountered a dilemma. In 1989 the Acid House scene had been represented by a yellow 'smiley face' and there were several for sale… yet it wasn't right. I didn't want a symbol attached to my jacket that actively *promoted* the drug and, alternatively, there were unhappy yellow badges with tongues protruding as if to say "arrh!" and that wasn't right either. Under the surface it is

48

microscopically possible that I admitted I had risked my sanity during those trips. The bizarre electrical taste in my teeth... the surface hallucinations of the Artex ceiling coming down in a blue/green shimmer of plaster... regularly saying "20,000 volts!" and *"everything's everywhere..."* yet it might also have generated thoughts that hadn't noticeably caused me harm, which may have taught me wisdom. Then I saw a badge that represented both sides. The little black in the white and the little white in the black of the supreme balance from a philosophy older than Christianity entitled: *Yin and Yang*. I plucked a medium sized badge off the board and stared at it. I had seen this before and had thought it an unimportant message within baseless chic. Seeing it again with open eyes, and an open mind, it was remarkable.

No doubt magnified by the *push-sub*-thoughts of interior *scu*, it seemed I was holding the key to grasping all of it. Registering its potential I saw that it expressed both slants of anything within the 'S' of a perfect balance - for example, there is a little man in a woman reflected by a little woman in a man - and it is blatantly structured to rotate. The direction of its rotation depends on whether you are looking at the underside of the symbol or the 'surface' that logic dictates runs clockwise. I turned the symbol round and round the wrong way and saw the essence of it flying to pieces. I applied it to L.S.D: on the large *black side* it can induce psychosis - with the small *white spot* in the black that it's very cheap and available for its potential: and reflected in the large *white side* is that you can learn a lot from it, maybe even <u>bypass</u> the wisdom acquired through years of natural experience – with the small *black spot* that whatever its financial cost won't change the fact that it is illegal. This application is a dusty approximation of an incomplete memory set. Of course, there maybe other costs, so many. I turned the symbol in the correct direction by its centralised pin and I was sold. The *Yin and Yang* looked entrancing and it had a wonderful potential, so I bought it. I took the badge back to Colchester knowing it would add new dimension to the conversations I shared with Tony. My friend and I explored our beliefs parked in the darkness amongst the arable farmland between Mersea and Colchester, passing joints each way in the car. We got high yet we could still lock our thoughts in lively discussion. That exotic smell filled our cocoon and music encouraged a sense of being annexed from civilisation. When the *Yin/Yang* is addressed properly, in terms of its reflectivity, it can be an excellent therapy that proves there is no reason for, or against, doing anything. A person can do anything they want to do metered according to levels of seriousness of their act - dictated by their moral values. "But these boundaries can be pushed forward", one of us said. The reply may have been: "If it doesn't hurt anyone else what the hell does it matter?" Tony and I were not afraid to get into real philosophy, our consciousnesses apparently on a par with each other. "There's a bit of death in life right, so it must mean... that there is a <u>little life in death</u>!"

For me this was more proof of re-incarnation as a working system. We were becoming free of the hooks and chains of paranoia and saw *karma* as the positive result of the spiral I mentioned in Chapter One. It is another issue of reflectivity that has a kind of death at both ends. Your movement on this spiral is dictated by wisdom garnered from experience, in slow steps, but a drug bypassing that process makes for huge jumps. At the top of the spiral you become happy in your knowledge – as content as though you have learned everything you have to know - and this is a representational 'death' after which if you are an Artist with a capital 'A' you offer up small bites of the secret with your recognised medium. And Tony and

I also believed that there was death at the bottom of this spiral, also, through a destroyed mind, suicide through the depression of that perception in reverse.

We were far "up, up, and away" from that horror, parked in East Mersea one night talking and sharing joints, a police car showed up. We were 'bang to rights', sitting in a grey cloud of dope smoke like aliens caught in an abandoned spaceship. Yet, strangely, the car just turned round and drove away. We saw this as a kind of divine licence to continue. One evening I was in a pub after smoking strong grass and the people drinking around me were on a totality different wavelength. I had a reality crisis, felt a separation from them (later in life I would call them 'beer-monsters') but then I stood with my back to the counter... and I saw these people were all apparently paranoid themselves and they hadn't touched any of that powerful weed! *Everybody is paranoid* so I thought. My inferiority complex reversed.

In the beginning of spring Tony and I seemed to have beaten paranoia and we were walking around safely free and feeling happy in our knowledge. I initiated a few little personal ceremonies when I was alone. I felt I might do something special for my 21st birthday on 12th March. At the flat I had told Migs "You're not an adult until you're twenty one!" We never wondered as to whether we had released ourselves from a natural aspect of life, dumped a 'defence mechanism' that we knew could be a part of everyone, but perhaps that's conjecture – thinking beyond the idea that everybody else was paranoid too may never have happened. With our mentalities become so beautifully different to that of society it could be said that Tony and I had become blissfully insane. But people have different opinions of what is "normal" and I've met a few who claim not to know what it means at all. That is a great cliché of psychiatry.

We went out again near my birthday. After these inner experiences everything had somehow changed between Tony and I. Our learning curves were no longer synchronised and as we tried to talk our points of view started rocketing off in opposing directions. It seemed neither of us could understand a single thing the other was saying. I expressed a theory that somehow we had become split into a *Yin-Yang* configuration. He drove me back to my parents and we went back to our own thoughts. I wasn't to see him again until after my birthday and then only twice before I was committed to a mental hospital.

At about ten o'clock on the night of March 11th I walked into the Mersea community centre intending later to absorb myself in a moment of midnight joy. I would dance on the beach, celebrate my 21st birthday under the moon to confirm my well being and immerse myself in a ceremony to validate the suspicion I felt, then, that I was some kind of a 'god'. With a pocket stereo in my coat loaded with an original cassette of *"Zoo Look"* by Jean Michel Jarre, the haunting album Tony and I had used to encourage our connection, I sat on a bar stool and ordered a drink. The man on duty that clear and unseasonably warm night let me know his birthday was on the 12th March also. Past being surprised by anything I suggested, with a slightly contrived casual amusement, that we exchange presents, and gave each other packets of nuts. I put mine away.

At half past eleven, I sat on the ground against the window of a shop selling books and art equipment, opposite the churchyard. I rolled a weak joint and felt the proximity of an epiphany in my learning curve, a delicious anticipation that I was soon to be fulfilled. I smoked only half of the joint. I was already ready for anything so just before twelve I walked around the corner onto Coast Road then down the concrete steps onto the beach where I found the water was washing up near the detritus that marked the high-tide line. At midnight I started playing the music. A chunky 'Magnox' power-station called Bradwell is about two miles away across the estuary from where I began. A full moon suspended at forty degrees directly over the station lit the beach with a pale mystery. Bradwell twinkled with lights and the stars above were arrayed yet muted by the plump moon with its unfathomable influences upon the blood and the oceans. I danced, and it was warm, still. I flowed with Jean's first song, a finesse of arms and fingers moving artfully like flamenco, and I was alone, free to communicate myself unseen by anyone but the lords above – it was an exquisite 'Now'...

Like a wind blowing across the surface of a dusty planet, the first track expresses well the spirit of Barker's 'un-belonging', with the cries of an alien creature howling far away in the distance for another of itself. An aspect deep inside the music was a noise like a relentlessly turning machine. I thought of a gigantic *Ying-Yang* engine, imagined it rotating in deep space, saw the image of it overlaid on the stars to the top left of Bradwell and the moon suspended over the twin monoliths of its roofs. Near the water I drew the symbol in the sand and tore open the packet of nuts. I sprinkled them onto it as an offering to Godly Force, and bowed as I have done sometimes when leaving churches – as courtiers used to leave the presence of their monarch – I bowed while pacing backwards. Then, as an older man who has tasted something else, something of the 'Beyond' and made more than I had been because of it, I walked back to the house knowing it was a place in which I no longer belonged. I climbed under my duvet and slept like the dead.

The *Nightbreed Chronicles* carried me the rest of the way into madness. I was hospitalised a week after that night and I hadn't even seen the film! In the *Chronicles* I began to recognise members of my own family: 'Lizzie B', also known as 'Miss Sheer 1944', 'Brain Pan Betty', "The Gully Mistress" and other names, that she is "aspiring transparency", and my mum's name is Liz. She was born in 1944 and I was a little angry Barker had referred to her with such insults. Another creature is to be seen wearing the 'price' of looking for a moment into my reality, is named 'Frick', my earthly father so I thought then, his face stretched during the moment he shied away from that vision. And I felt, looking upon the page, that Frick could also mean "Fuck Rick". My elder sister's character was "Radinka", who because of the damage I caused our family (and my radiated energy) was described as "the woman who sees only the past". And my younger sister (within the book the daughter of a Nightbreed woman, the exquisite Rachel) is called Babette, with curly blonde hair that I remember thinking she would have looked alike the girl in the photograph when it had been taken. Obviously in the name "Babette" is "Baby Boone".

It became obvious to me that many of the monsters to be seen were Barker's friends, actors who weren't quite acting, and given secret recognition. Telepaths he had 'bought off' with parts to play in a film that had the latent possibility its fiction could pour itself into the real world. And there were other psychological conditions that may never have seemed as palatable as being Barker's "Cabal". The priest called "Ashbury", made *Nightbreed* also, whose name suggests a religiously stubborn insanity about never enjoying a cigarette again; the loved-up feeling of chocolate represented by the three pristine white babies of a character called 'Chocolat'; 'Kinski', who took a drug which could change his features and drifted away staring at the night sky on the high the drug induced so his face took the form of a crescent moon – which I thought referred to the Russian actress I had found pretty named Nastassia Kinski. "Kolka Three Flies": a creature that never washed. "Kex": young pub violent beer monsters. "The Thrall": who had taken and pushed every drug he could get down his neck and ended up a prophet after disintegrating himself into a mess of legs and arms botched together like a wobbly shit pile. "Decker", the insane psychiatrist who I felt represented someone in reality that destroyed people with drug prescriptions rather than knives. "Pesoa the Pale": who's name is very similar to a brand of contact lens I used to use, far off at the exhausted ending of the story, a beaten man with one eye issuing three 'dire prophesies' and Boone's best friend in the plot who had first confirmed the directions to *Midian*, the ex-actor "Narcis".
People in the public, 'Naturals' who have a similar appearance to celebrities may be 'a chip off the old block'. The celebrity is the *originator*, at the top of a pyramid of their kind, at the apex of hundreds of others diluting towards the base. The suggestion that there maybe a finite number of similar features connecting types of people opens the forum for some insane debate - angels fighting a war for heaven, tribal telepathy war, aliens fighting for the Earth - every far-

out theory you can be punished for believing. So where was *Lori*?

Where was my beautiful lover to be? Through *Scu* driven perception I saw the *Nightbreed* monsters as mostly all having brown eyes - my colour, except for hers. Rather than the originator I was more likely to meet a girl lower on her 'pyramid'. In early 1990 I thought if I wanted to be Lori's man I would have to take on *Cabal* as prophesy. For a powerful example, in the beginning of the film Decker had shown a sheaf of photographs to his patient, frames of people Boone had allegedly killed - and every single picture in *The Nightbreed Chronicles* has a serrated edge. Tearing them out neatly and handing them to people corresponding to the characters in my environs seems to be a part of the book's design. These 'Naturals' would have their realities changed so utterly, if they actually *believed*, they would have been metaphorically 'killed' matching Boone's description of being 'a trampler and a transformer'. Then, once collected, the photographs could be poured over my psychiatrist's desk exactly like in the film!

A loose definition of the word *Cabal* describes a conspiracy, usually of four people, uninteresting until I learnt of the meaning of the fifth. In an encyclopaedia that probably hadn't been opened for years I read that some centuries ago there had reined an English king who had found himself stuck between four great tribal leaders. He had been surrounded by warlords of the North, South, East and West, and he had balanced them from the centre, juggled them, and successfully. He had been the fifth, played them off against each other and lived to reign to a grand old age. I hated the concept of my flesh family in those days so I took on board grander relations: Sean Connery, as my father, Kate Bush, my mother and Enya
Brennan, my sister: and Clive Barker, who knows? Being stuck in the midst of these Artists, more specifically, being in the middle of the *forces* that they represent from the centre was a nightmare that did not occur to me immediately. Details would change.

Enemy sub-thought that I could never accept was that the *Cabal* position had engendered the title of Barker's novella of "Hellraiser" – called *The Hellbound Heart*. I felt that if this was true, if it was to be *my heart* going to hell, anyway, there wouldn't have been any point to doing *any* of it. However there are more traps in Barker's work than you can poke a wooden stake at. And now, writing of this from time's leading edge, I'm still here and still alive twelve years later and the war may draw to a quiet and mostly uneventful end.

In the second week of March, between my birthday and being committed to hospital, Robert visited me at my parent's house. He had brought with him a cassette of a new album called *"Violator"* by Depeche Mode, which I thought he had been playing to test me, to assess my light and darkness. But I had thought that some of it was darkly brilliant! The songs were like a boat with drum beats carrying ghosts smoothly along a rushing black river. With my pocket stereo I listened to "World in my eyes" and "Enjoy the Silence" and it could be said that this album became the musical essence of early 1990 – along with *"The Dark Side of the Moon"* by Pink Floyd. I haven't seen Robert again more than once ever since.

The last tussle I had with Tony was around March 15th when one of us had phoned the other. I went up to his mother's on Gun Fleet Close, where Tony had ushered me upstairs. He took out a slip of yellow paper and I could tell this was another Big One. No discussion. It was about verification. "I'm not gay, right?" he said: "Take my hand!" I did. "Now look in my eyes." His hand was warm and heavy, and I started falling into his eyes. Our pupils would logically have opened up like gates and I would learn seven years later that this is called 'eye-diving'. I peered into him like something I had seen before, in the shopping precinct long ago, but much more affecting like I was on a quiet railway moving between realties with a distant prickling. And his hand felt apocryphal, a kind of flimsy unimportant parallel to his soul. This flesh machine was just a vehicle to carry around his spirit. Tony withdrew his hand and unfolded the piece of yellow paper.

He exclaimed "*It's got a name*! It's called KISS! – *Keep It Simple Stupid*... look at this!" He showed me what had been handwritten on his note, which I assumed was from someone he knew at work. "Dear Tony – well done! *KISS*." I was stunned. Not only was there a machination of Artists dripping secrets to society – beyond the reach of press or politics (with mental illness the scapegoat of telepathy) – but there was also a conspiracy of the public, for people living in a linked understanding of themselves. Not the mind-life of telepaths but a community of equal parts in a commonly shared reality, without distance, a friend's initiation encouraging his adept into the fold. And, of course, it magnified my psychosis about Barker... but before I went to hospital there were a couple more revelations of which I must tell.

At the flat I had made a loose friendship with a man named Tim Herring. He had a pronounced pattern on his forehead when he frowned that looked like a 'gate'. With *push-subs* I associated that this enabled him the capability to vampire energy or air like the creature Peloquin, and the man actually told me that his tribe were called *the "Hoovids"*. He was my age and liked his illicit drugs. It was clear we had been chasing for gold up some of the same beanstalks but had wound up quite different. Tim had almost no possessions, a long ponytail, and the calmness of the enlightened. He was a well-read man who was comfortable with himself and his own secrets. On the afternoon before the night of the British Association of Film and Television Awards (known as the BAFTAs, around March 16th 1990) I went into Colchester with him and we snorted some amphetamine 'speed' bought from a pub. For me, then, it was the first time. It didn't seem to do much, yet judging by my mentality during the night that followed it must have caused a massive reaction in brain chemistry – if you'll excuse the cheapness of this – it was like an "award leading to a ward"!

I sat in the lounge watching the BAFTAs with my parents and I had floating sensations, felt something welling up within me close to godhood. I was full of pride for a future not yet begun, proud ahead of time for things I hadn't done yet. I was comfortable knowing that through progressive logic, from being a "Hero of the Night" I was therefore the Anti-Christ figure in this unfolding drama yet paradoxically not a bad man. That was a severe misdirection by Barker. He had awoken a part of me, a knowledge that held no terror for me then, more like a kind of 'punch drunk' amazement. A Princess took to the stage while I was 'spanning out', and I knew that all Artist's could feel it, my radiated energy. I can remember two sentences she said in particular: "We all know the one about Barkers and hares. This is a very great moment for Art..." and then they played a song with the lyrics: "Every breath you take, every claim you stake, every step you take I'll be watching you..." by a band called *The Police*. This was enough.

I told my folks I was a god. My mother told me to take a bath. I went up and drew the water. That night I was so high I saw planets and galaxies in the bubbles and manipulated a black universe in the tub. I smoked a Marlboro and felt utterly huge, pressed the Jacuzzi switch so the black surface filled with white bubbles and felt that with the touch of a button I had made an inverted universe! – Soon after I had a hellish experience in another bathroom, in an empty tub, with a spider crawling all over me. I had gone on a massive bad trip with shower-head tap-twists of temperature, from 'freezing' to 'boiling' and I was yelling, groaned loudly and muttered until my mother showed up and shouted "what's the matter?" I dried off. This event has since caused the Enemy to propose that my soul came from a spider but they are notorious liars and *attack scu* are, if nothing else, opportunists.

Later during the day Tony had inducted me into *KISS*. I ran back to Gun Fleet Close carrying a hardback edition of *The First Book of the Art,* or maybe just the dust jacket. My circumstances were so unique that I felt *KISS* was beneath me. I wanted to impress upon Tony that there were other related interests to be seen here if you just scrape the earth off the bones... yet maybe revealing the skeleton of a monster called <u>psychosis</u> that was coming alive to bite my head off and swallow it like a tablet of medication. To me it was clear from the cover of *"The 1st Book of the Art"* that there were situations rolling and intertwining here that were simply huge. I needed to be understood, so I showed this art to Tony's mother and it seemed that she grasped a few things I didn't. She looked upset and asked piercingly: "Have you ever been in a mental hospital?" Then she said: "<u>Don't</u> go *there*!" but this imperative may have referred less to matters of geography and more to the possibility that she saw me as blind man about to walk off a cliff. But I had discovered there was magic in the world, real Magic, and the promise of adventure. I had been awakened and given purpose, guided by the prophecy of a master. I was going all the way.

CHAPTER FOUR: *Hospital Part One*

18th March was a beautiful day for such a grim appointment. Believing by then that I was Boone, not overtly evil, yet paradoxically the Anti-Christ, the community mental health team and my family's GP Doctor Marshall interviewed me in my parent's garden. I stood before them in the afternoon of a warm sun wearing black denim, a black tank top, and a studded leather belt. They asked me if I would take off my mirror glasses but I said "no" and told them that when they looked at me I wanted them to see themselves. I was ready for the prophecy to begin. That was intoxicating in itself, so I rapidly volunteered for treatment. Evening saw me pack some things, including the *Nightbreed Chronicles* for anyone I met corresponding to its characters, and I was driven by my father to Severalls Hospital in Colchester.

I was admitted onto a ward with two wings, a Victorian psychotic exercise yard called Myland Court.
It had a games room with a half sized snooker table, a cafeteria serving food that I would find tasted like paper because of all the excitement between meals, a patient's kitchen; a sitting room with a large bay window and a TV that seemed to be powered by cigarette smoke instead of electricity. It was divided at night into the East wing for women, the West wing for men. The borders were broken during the day but I had little interest in sex.

My perception was alive there, and dark. Greased with a sprinkling of black miracles my unsociable situation became palatable through my oblivious interaction with the ward. I looked back on those days as being an adventure: yet Barker, satisfying in this example his lust for total power, had driven me utterly out of control. I had walked around outside picking up bits and pieces of meaningless crap as if I had no brain of my own – but a headless chicken doesn't run about for very long. I unpacked my things and during the second night I went through an event like nothing I had ever experienced before, a bizarre 'awakening'.

My head began sparkling with a creeping ache. I was being changed, believed that for every Artist who had ever died one cell was waking up in my brain. I crawled in the night, groaning around the corridors. I knew it wasn't a 'normal' headache and I had to ask one of the staff for some sticky back Celotape to seal my eyes shut so I could get some sleep. Later on, I would call this a 'Tip' from Barker to myself, a forest fire sweeping through my skull as the bones behind my face softened and altered. I never got the Celotape or hardly slept.

The pain diminished as the sun rose. I discovered the outer orbital lobes of my skull on the extreme edges of my eye sockets had a growth of new bone; hard, triangular, protrusions. As I looked into a Mirror, I wrinkled my forehead towards the top of my nose: and the skin there became a succession of triangles pointing down at an angle on each side that looked angry. I wrinkled my forehead upwards and eight or nine bars appeared folded into the skin. I wrinkled toward my nose horizontally and saw the shape of a Gate with three bars above it – like Tim's forehead 'signature' as I was beginning to think of the phenomena. I considered both the expressional wrinkles of Actors and Actresses, and also of the patterns of grooves and ridges in the face in the photograph of Boone in his bestial state. This was hard proof. And I also thought about *The Books of Blood* particularly Barker's idea of escaping your hell by tricking your responsibility onto someone else's shoulders…

I took a side room near the ward's public telephone to write myself, as though it was an office. It was an occupation that I intended calling the *Second Book of the Art,* based on the fiction of the first being educated by the awareness of my sequel as 'reality', a favourite theme of mine, obviously!   I wanted to write of skills I was just beginning to grasp. How to 'buddy energy' around to each other (which in my case was with cigarettes) or how to reach behind you and locate objects without seeing those (1990!). How to 'Air-Attack' with deep breaths from the lower middle rib cage area, after a lock-on to the target (face to face / on a scu-line / or perhaps with a photograph) which was Peloquin's talent. It was his weapon to cause tiredness (oxygen withdrawal) or the panic of qualming (energy withdrawal) and I assisted my own assaults with hard-core trance music in my headphones and by sucking Halls Extra Strong menthol lozenges in a silver and black packet. I hardly wrote a page about this mind-life. I figured the *Third Book of the Art* would write itself.

My room was numbered 102, between the medication room and seclusion room 101. It felt like a prison cell in a library with its essence of beginnings and quietness and dusty wood. Psychiatric drugs were an anathema to me. The first dose ever given to a new patient always brings them rudely crashing back to their difficult new situation. The staff didn't give me any for two or three days while they were getting the measure of me. I asked my Key Nurse if Decker was about. "No Deckers here Richard, it's an asylum you know? A safe place." Later I could have told her that the other definition of that word was accurate also. The entire place had a lot of people who were a few orange segments short of a fruit salad, including some of the staff. It was a challenge to know who were actually the nurses and who were the patients, and I lapped it up!

When my prescription began, four nurses applied an amber liquid to me in a beaker. I learned later it was a 'cosh' called Chlorpromazine. They insinuated it was poison. Two men and two women stood in pairs looking at me silently with eyes I perceived to be all brown. I broke the silence. "Who the Hell is you people?" And they told me they were the Four Horses of the Apocalypse, and (approximately) that I was no longer 'useful' to the cause. A nurse named Marcus sat with me after the others had gone, making sure I ate a tuna salad, which I thought was my last meal. Then he tied my shoelaces, handed me the beaker of liquid, and told me I would 'sleep' soon. I drank it thinking the Horses were on their way, already, to the four corners of the Earth. It was the first time of many that I accepted death. Although telepaths understand the essence of a Quiddity Afterlife I knew nothing of it then – just Tim's theory that "heaven is whatever you want it to be" which is correct had I only been able to understand its workings and affect. I was wearing only one contact lens at the time, and, about to die, I popped it out and chewed it up. I spat it onto the floor then lay on my back waiting for heart to slow, to slow and stop; or burst, or go crazy with arrhythmia or something. Yet the beat went on, and I left the room alive.

An aspect of psychosis, which is exciting, is to have your beliefs verified by people you've never met before. I knew about 'grids' from movies like Terminator and the grid I'd seen at the flat on Mersea during one of those calmer evenings: The 'fencing mask' of red dots within red equilateral triangles that I had hallucinated for a moment, and never since. I concluded it was the base framework underlying visual registry, and maybe another kind of 'signature'. I suspected that there also existed a Battle Grid seen, I thought then, through the left eye. Later I gathered a conflicting idea that the soul sees through the left eye and the machinery of bodies look through the right. Check the different eyes of your friends and family to see this for yourself! Even in the portraits of Grand Masters you will rarely see eyes painted symmetrically in a painting. A 'BAFTA' award has the right eye open and the left closed. "If thine right eye offends thee, pluck it out," the Good Book says. The T-101 terminator in the movie did just that. And my grid, so I thought, was sensed in the left eye because I was right eye dominant then and more comfortable seeing that way.

I was talking to a student nurse, another Tim, of small secrets such as the fact that every bar code in British shops is divided into segments by three 6s. And another, that the 999 telephone number of the British Police can make the number 666 of The Beast if turned upside down, when I noticed one of

his eyes was of a darker colour than the other. He told me he was wearing a red-tinted contact lens in his left eye. I assumed it was for him to 'feel' the extra sense of his visual instincts – a nurse (!) who had escorted me to the main building, once, and had shown me his meagre pay cheque in a way that had seemed slightly embarrassed, as if he had felt the need to apologise because he was on the other side, 'with them'. I told him I didn't need a red lens because I already have a benign 'nevus', a small red spot in my left eye, which has a strong prescription of a feeble focal length of about four inches!   I could take out either lens. This facility lent me a divided up way of seeing things with a weird simultaneity that created the sense of having the instincts of a machine. I don't remember what else Tim the nurse and I talked about. We most likely fed each other with other rabid facts.

To move into a wider world I needed to sacrifice my past so I pushed my soft blue pillowcase into the throat of an ashtray in the TV room. A few days later it re-appeared back on my bed, folded neatly and washed, and I never knew who had done it. I was once asked a question in Myland Court by a hard looking patient that had plasters on his wrists, which appeared slim enough to signal his wounds would be soon be healed, perhaps then an unfinished thought. The man had asked: "Do you see bubbles, or grids?" And I was fascinated and replied. Then, of course, I had to ask him what the 'bubbles' were but he was evasive. He said something like: "You don't want to know. Bubbles burst." We hung out a little and he unexpectedly punched someone in the patients' kitchen who had given me trouble. The man told me he was going to Germany soon – a few days later he was gone.

I used to go running through the hospital grounds driven by music like *"On the Run"* by Pink Floyd. I had thought their *Dark Side of the Moon* album was about anyone in the previous two and a half decades who had thought they were me! "I've been mad for fucking years, absolutely years," so the lyrics go. The band must have had one of the worst and maddest postbags in history: "Lethal today gone tomorrow that's me!" I listened to Depeche Mode as well, and Snap's *The Power* during jogging or Air-Attack, and I exercised so I could be fit for 'the end' during which, in some dark October in the long future, I would go on my own 'run'. I concealed the *Nightbreed Chronicles* in the woods beneath a 'lay tree' most likely because of a *push-sub* that it wasn't safe in my room.

Another student nurse in Myland Court, called Heather, was one of the most beautiful women I ever met. She told me she was a black belt in Kick Boxing and I saw no reason not to believe her. With black hair and deep blue eyes revealing a kind of tired cynicism, Heather had a stunning womanly shape in revealing black clothes; extraordinary, a story all to herself, and I wished her to be my Lori. We spoke little at first. I wanted her to think of me as a mystery but I caught her eye sometimes like there were bolts of lightning flashing between us. One afternoon I showed her Barker's book. We might have sat together on that lost tree as I watched her wondering upon this intimacy, but she dismissed being Lori. I fingered a few pages along and found the character called 'Rachel' whose physical beauty was frowned upon by other *Nightbreed*. "A prisoner of her own symmetry" as it was written... and perhaps this exquisite student had also been disadvantaged by her loveliness, particularly in the job she was being trained for. I showed her Murray Close's photograph of 'Rachel' and Heather neither confirmed nor denied any connection with herself. Yet she had looked, briefly, as though there might be other things going on under her professional patina challenging me to accept the unspoken possibility of her agreement.

I believed telepathy was rife. I also believed that many people knew of me, so, in spite of this meaning a 'safe place' was necessary. I actually escaped twice. One night I bedded down in a trailer on a building site and the business cards that I found in a desk drawer were secret code. Another time, I ran out into busy traffic and stole a whole case of milk off the back of a van. Later, I thought I could buy a bus ticket to Mersea for 11 pence and after I was kicked off it, I decided to go there on foot. So I walked and walked for over eight miles and when I arrived home my Dad drove me back to the ward within half an hour. Wandering around the nearby industrial estate I found a red Ferrari with the number plate "WAR" that I thought I could buy for Monopoly money. I believed that the 0898 sex lines were mind-to-mind numbers. All of this and more, *sub-thoughts* being pushed into the mind of a man that barely had any faculty of reason left. Just a psychoses flourishing within me that made me believe all of it was true because I thought I was too intelligent to really be 'mentally ill'.

Some nights I wished and believed that I was 'mind-melting' with the raven-haired Heather. Sometimes I took myself in hand in the soft darkness. I was beginning to think of her as having a false 'tag' for her own protection. Deep down, I was thinking that 'Heather' was not the name written on her driver's licence: her name was Rachel, same as the *Nightbreed* character. But the biggest drawback of all was the rules that prevented our connection: she was a nurse and I was a patient.

I played snooker. I used to believe the colours were metaphorical, that the ancients who had conceived the game had known exactly how the Armageddon thing was going to pan out. "Helicopters and guns!" I shouted. "London to Oslo in 15 minutes!" I played snooker with the beautiful nurse, also, two or three times. "I always have trouble getting the pink down," I'd told her – meaning potting a girlfriend at 'the end' before the black ball. It was a weird exclamation and could have been assimilated by individual patients in many ways. That is how everything can get worse. We uttered unintelligible non-sequesters in the *Now* and other patients heard these and assimilated them into their own belief systems, dragging them into deeper illness. If anyone could be blamed for a similar tactic it was in part down to the methods of the staff. I later learnt that 'The Four Nurses of the Apocalypse" might have been known as a 'Rapid Access Team', nursing that suppressed new patients by feeding them wind-ups in order to discover the extent of their illness and what it is made of. If you reckon that sounds OK you just remember the acting of those nurses tricked me into thinking I was going to die. Bastards.

I bravely 'palmed' masses of my prescription. Standing before the drug trolley you are given a beaker of water with which to swallow the tablets. It is a beaker so tiny it feels like a statement that you are being denied access to purity in direct contrast to the substances. I was relaxed when the staff handed me mine because I had a cigarette before medication time. I hid the tablets under my tongue. One of the staff, a woman with a face that wrinkled up like a weasel when she was defending her satisfaction, sometimes made "I smell something!" sniffing noises. If she did do this to induce paranoia it probably worked because I thought she was a referring to my Marlboros, which I was considering giving up.

Heather (or 'Rachel') said: "Come on Rich, time to get your 'meds'" to me, two or three times. She actually said 'meds'. It really hurt. I chucked the pills behind my wardrobe until March 31st when I had weekend leave in West Mersea. I got back on April 1st when a nurse called Vicky, one of the Horses, said that they'd found those discarded tablets so I wasn't allowed pills anymore. A Welsh nurse and I had been on the floor, sitting against the wall of room 102, once, and he told me then: *"You've already done it,"* a reference to cycles? The new prescription of Chlorpromazine was to be applied 'in liquid suspension' in beakers with other stuff called *Procyclodine* to cope with the confusing issue of side-affects. But there was still a lot of fight left in me.

Following 'April Fool's Day' I developed a new routine. I got out of bed and went down early to the cafeteria and collected a bowl of dry cereal, and a cup of cool milk, two pieces of dry toast on a plate, and butter. I used to hide them in my room then go back down and drink half a cup of coffee before medication time. I swallowed the beaker of foul fluid, asked for the shower room to be opened and a towel. Next, I stuck a toothbrush down my throat in the shower and 'puked up' as much of it as I could. Then I dried off, got dressed, and casually ate breakfast in my room. The student nurse Tim once gave me my towel in the morning. It had been NHS towel with pale stripes of red made lacklustre from excess washing. He had said that the colour was "to match the red in your eyes." I had thought then it had been said because I was straining my eyes puking up in the shower. Later I realised he was talking about our eyes – the eyes of the grid. I did see a Battle Grid, on *one occasion* but there were other ways to fight.

One night in bed I had been trying to have a mind-melt with my beloved when another nurse creaked open the door of 102 and interrupted me with a torch. I didn't much care if he had just been doing his job. I popped a strong menthol lozenge into my mouth set my stereo playing *Snap*, and Air-Attacked him. I walked past the Nurses Station a moment later to see if there had been any damage. I looked through the window and saw him staring back at me with an expression on his sallow exhausted face that told the entire story. Wide disbelieving eyes being overcome by the intensity in my own; all greys and haggard skin, yet he would have forgotten all about it within a week, supposing it had even happened! I churned out my own force like telepath's do, which should produce the affect of charisma, but mine was being output *in reverse* through the base-control-set. At a subconscious level this would most likely have scared good people away.

Jason, the young man who had bitten out half of his tongue because of an over-dose of Haliperidol had been strutting around the TV room one afternoon like a peacock saying he was Flash Gordon and I was Ming "The Merciless". So I Air-Attacked him also. I have kept in loose contact with Jason since and he has told me the result of this withdrawal recently.

When he had been bristling up to me I engaged *Snap* with full menthol and sucked in with gestures of hauling rope. I was adventuring...

He told me 12 years later that at the time he had hallucinated a giant mosquito on the TV room carpet. Whether I had the capability to Air Attack after 'The Tip' – and not before – I don't know. Yet here at least is some proof that such a weapon works. Out there are some people that in comparison to my feeble vacuuming can engage fifty-foot diameter nuclear-powered wind tunnels, if you know what I mean? Barker's associates: *His soldiers.*

The first time I was ever dragged back into a ward by the staff was spectacular. I went through a bay window in the television room like an express train. One moment I was absently examining the flimsy wood and the flaky paint as though it had been composed of paper-mache and the next I was putting my boot through it. To anyone gently catching some T.V it must have sounded like a bomb going off. Shards of wood and glass crashed onto the cement as I ducked through the huge hole and started to run across the road onto the grass with grids blazing – a yellow Battle Grid of moving crosses and perhaps numbers – that I only ever saw at this moment. If it wasn't the *scu* high-jacking my Imager, I was seeing the last vestiges of ancient redundant equipment. The Battle Grid may have been an echo of a material plane war that good people had lost long ago. Four, maybe five, nurses dragged me back to my room where they yanked my trousers down half way. They jabbed me with sedatives so hard one of my legs ached for hours. I might have been aware, vaguely, that 'Heather' was not one of them. That was good.

Wanting to approach her surreptitiously I left a cassette cover of an album called "The Hurting", by *Tears for Fears*, under a wiper on the windscreen of her car. It has a picture of a little boy on it and I underlined the word "Hurting". One afternoon, I walked into the cafeteria attracted to talking. There was no meal being served and I was not hungry for anything except a cigarette (I'd kicked the shit out of the habit because I was emitting too much energy – without knowing at that time that the exacerbated withdrawal of interior *scu* was going to kick the shit out of me) – and, of course, there was my hunger for her. "I dreamt my boyfriend shot me in the head with a gun," she had said to her captive audience, and I had thought the dream indicated me. I beseeched her, cried out "*Rachel, Rachel*, don't say that!" and ran. At the top of a set of stairs I found my way barred by a locked door. When she caught up with me, she asked: "*how did you know my name is Rachel?*" and that had been amazing. I liked to think our relationship changed then.

She gave me the local telephone number of her martial arts teacher, who went by the name Reza. The hero's best friend in the prophecy is called "Narcis", which is as phonetically similar to Reza as scissors are to razors. Shortly before my release I phoned him and the call was received by Rachel who passed me to him. Thus, I thought he may have been her boyfriend. He asked me: "Do you want to escape?!!" I think that he had asked this because it tallies with my breathless answer. I *distinctly recall* replying: "No, thank you, I always wanted to just walk out of here." After a journey of finding middle class men needing code words and other bizarre incidents, I met Reza at his house in Woodrush End. He wanted me call him "Ceephoo" – master – but it hadn't seemed right. He also told me to "give up the drugs" and I hated drugs so I saw him this one time only. Around April 20th 1990, I did just "walk out". I was discharged from the ward and walked to my father's car with a suitcase in one hand and a bottle of Chlorpromazine in the other. I left there *far* crazier than when I had been admitted and I hadn't even kissed my Lori. I tried to create that opportunity by returning to Severalls a free man, three weeks later, but I never saw her again.

I worried my family deeply and regularly. My sister Ellie was away one night so I stayed in her breezy room, which had been Dad's original office. I was very ill and I didn't sleep until dawn. In the florescent light in the early hours of the night I started crawling over Ellie's carpet, pressing my fingertips into it, a blue and green silk 'weaveworld'. I thought that many Artists worked with such carpets to ease telepathy by using the patterns and swirls like a telephone exchange. A desire to make love with the West forces of purity and water came over me. In my imagination I envisaged a room on board a ship called the 'Ephemeris' (Barker's name for the islands in *Quiddity*), which had a bedroom with perhaps a four-poster in rich reds of lush velvet. The deed became masturbation on my sister's 'weaveworld' with an Irish lady, a matter of commitment and superstition. The carpet levied an importance upon the act and broadcast the significance of the woman I chose.

I sneaked in a cigarette afterwards and burnt a hole with it into the centre of the carpet that Barker's mythical writing calls "the Gyre". I balanced an egg-shaped soap on the hole. This represented the pregnancy of new life, and perhaps those other 'sisters' in hospitals that you can never kiss or cuddle. I came out of the dark went down into the cool freshness of the garden's first sun kiss. It smelt of clean earth and wet grass. I felt kind of smug about the progress of my adventures and the dawn was bright compared to the furtive hours I had spent upstairs lost in myself. Bird song heralded the new day and I listened to them twittering as if through a black curtain to an orchestra of tiny beaks. I went back upstairs.

In modern telepath language there is another meaning for the word *"Reach"*. It is engineered by a part of many telepath's brains called a *"Reacher"* for <u>divining extra-sensory facts</u> *that* time can evolve. Reaches are sometimes confirmed by a *"verifier"* or by a percentage likelihood that I was to call an *"estimator"*. Whether this is a 'verbally contagious' benign tumour or the resurgence of a primordial ability is moot – as human beings we rarely use over a quarter of our brains capability in a lifetime. I went on some huge benders of discovery, in those days, but I didn't know it was called *'reaching'* until seven years had passed. In the first month of 1997 that word was said to me a lot.

In 1990 a massive discovery developed in a round shaving mirror. It was cracked in three places lying on my duvet and I *reached* with the equivalent effect of zooming out and out. I placed mints on the glass (some stuck together) that somehow linked the thirds representing metaphysical areas known as *'vicinities'*. I don't remember if our own universe took up much room in the mirror but it was laid on my duvet that had a pattern which looked like a gigantic 'time grid'. That other comparably small structure of the universe was powered by a clove. For many decades people had pushed cloves into an orange to make an air-freshener, and that clove I plugged into the mirror's frame represented the unifying power linking *vicinities* and dimensions: the force of telepathy. Yet, I believed nevertheless that telepathy had no influence on the unimaginably huge 'time grid' outside it. This was exciting yet the description doesn't even *touch* the perfection I grasped when I photographed it.

On a Channel Four show, in 1989, I had seen Barker saying: "Now here are my feet." So I took B&W photos of my own because of his barely concealed *"kiss my feet"* metaphor, which had aroused anger and envy. There had been tantalising glimpses of *Nightbreed* SFX on the screen but crushed by concepts I was soon to spend over ten weeks in an Intensive Care Unit because of books about a movie that I hadn't even seen... I lost that roll of strange film but it's doubtful I would have understood the images on it if I hadn't. During the illusion of 'freedom' before my second admission my illness was like a motorcycle crashing through a forest. Moving in the 'Now', without intentionality, with questions answered and verifications witnessed. My radiation of mind-altering energy was going to create a 'Palomo Grove' event, a practise apocalypse on Mersea that would riot the tiny

Island into thrown fragments and smoke after which the world would never be the same.

I played a game of pool with the Greek Cypriot owner of the White Hart pub opposite the church. Many of his customers were rolling in the isles. To avoid aggravating their drunkenness I sometimes decided to *suck the energy out of myself!* There seemed to be an exaggerated importance to the game and I beat him. Then I asked: "Do you see bubbles or grids?" and he replied: "Bubbles." And I said: "Incredible isn't it? Bubbles aren't so good." "Why not?" / "Because bubbles burst." That was more or less how it went. Walking through the earthy green of a spring afternoon in Friday Woods I heard a sound that was unmistakable after seeing so many action films. It was the noise of someone amongst the trees firing a machine-gun. I walked into a clearing in the forest where I saw people, chaperoned by soldiers, firing blank rounds – clearly mentally disabled people with difficulties such as Downs Syndrome – and I was suspicious. It looked to me more like an experiment than a day out to the woods. On a side table were drinks and a soldier amiably gave me a cup of orange juice. I drank it and left, wondering what the hell the military thought it was doing.

At the side counter in the smell of ale in the West Mersea Yacht Club I waited for a man my Dad had told me was ex-Army. He was the manager. I came prepared with stickers from the chandlery down the road because I was worried that the military, who I believed 'knew' of me, should have a presence at the place my Dad attended so often. Aligned to the colours Red and Blue I also believed that the police would fight the army at 'the end', which meant that I distrusted the man and I wanted my position made clear. I stuck a *Marine-Watch* Police sticker to the bar furniture of a beer keg facing him on the counter, and the man came over to me. He saw the sticker and he looked like he was on a 'sacrificial pitch' ready to move beyond whatever theory with which he had come equipped. He read the words *'Marine Watch'* and nodded. Without a single smile between us during the exchange, I asked him: "Do you believe in telepathy?" and he closed his eyes, for a brief moment then said: *"Snow"*. I hadn't expected this, hadn't thought of 'broadcasting', but it was another revelatory moment.

The 'Palomo Grove' / Mersea Island apocalypse was due on the next full moon. It would be an event with connections to *The Stand,* by Stephen King – a masterful novel about the separation of two groups of people that had survived a bacteriological Armageddon, and this separation would become reality on a small scale. They would gather in two locations, the Blue group would meet at a newsagents (I suppose meeting outside the Police station would have been more apt) and the Red group would gather at a beachfront café called "Two Sugars," where I had seen a sticker in there, amongst dozens of others adhered to the outside of the counter, of a Ying Yang symbol with the words "Armalite Pro-life" written around it. The Army again, so I thought – maybe a whole division!

The quarter moon was waxing towards the cusp. My father wanted to take me to look around a private mental health unit: a Priory Group hospital, near Bromley, in Kent. I asked him "Is this place like an artists retreat?" and he said 'yes' but he probably mumbled it into a diaphanous white lie. The place is called Hayse Grove and I really didn't want to even look at it. In spite of a massive vacuum assault of my dad's energy on the way, with "Hurricane Mints", he drove us there unerringly and escorted me through to reception. The garden wasn't big but the cafeteria looked more like a restaurant. I also grasped that the place was drug-intensive, new admissions probably 'coshed' hard.

Standing beside me in front of a huge wooden octagonal desk (that served the I.C.U on one half and the reception on the other) was a little girl of about six. She was looking at me, then pulled at her mother's skirts, and asked her:

"Mummy is that the man who is going to turn Night into Day?"

Back on Mersea I stumbled across a BBC play called "Plato not NATO" broadcast on Radio Four. It mentioned a community centre, and gatherings of old people, and it seemed to be a guide to the incident fast approaching the Island. I wanted to turn Migs' flat into our own *Midian* and decorate it with bizarre graffiti and a green door and mystical paintings. I stole a map from the kitchen notice board in Tim Herring's parents' place when I had knocked on the door of an empty house. It was a map of Mersea, which had many odd coloured scribbles and markings in different areas that was blatantly secret cipher. Tim was a chip off Peloquin's old block – he *knew* – and that huge *'Hoovid'* box of an 'Air Qualm' gate on his forehead often comforted me with its undeniable physical truth. Tim later told me that the map I had taken hadn't been code at all, just a diagram of where his family and friends had been living!

I felt exposed then, perhaps in danger, because of my radiation of energy. If this output had indeed been reversed then the risks were likely to have been real. I strengthened my resolve not to smoke again and considered giving up caffeine also – dropping coffee like dropping off a tall building. On the threshold of moving to Mig's flat one night in the cold rain, my mother and I stood facing each other in the darkness at the front gate of High Acre. She prayed, so she has told me about the event since, and I reacted by walking back into the house. The last sunset I was to see as a free man was over the arable farmland of Essex after I forced my father to drop me off in the countryside. I had left him without much choice. Passing a house with a VW Beetle in the garden I knocked on the door because the car had been green. I asked the man who answered for what I had thought was my principal of identification: soda water and an apple... I was eating it when he asked if my parents knew if I was alright. He leant me his mobile phone. I dialled the number and told whoever answered that they shouldn't worry, that I was OK.

Soon I was walking down a lane and the day was ending. A golden sun was sinking into clouds at the end of the fields. An augur was promised me in a landscape bathed in orange fire. The interior *scu's* 'Attention-Grab' found me needing to look into a farm building. I walked up a short path of dried mud or old cement through a door into a ramshackle barn that had shafts of orange spearing the drifting dust like lasers through the holes in the woodwork. But I didn't see anything pretty.

I just saw death: the choice of a rope hanging from a beam or a bottle that looked as though it was two thirds full of Scotch. I thought the whisky would cause me to unravel in a 'Tip' back to Barker and I stood there floundering in the increasing darkness, flummoxed for a time I was unaware of passing. Then I heard a car pull up. I investigated it. It was my parents.

They thought it was best that we drive back to the hospital. A pale moon climbed the sky while I sat in the backseat like a tongueless parrot, or arguing my case. They revealed that the bloke who'd given me the apple had recalled them using the re-dial facility on his mobile phone. As soon as I had left he had called them back and told them of the direction I'd been walking in and my obvious mental instability. The 50%/50% moon got higher. My father drove us along the roads while we talked in bits of meanings like shrapnel. It had been a 'cusp' moon, it seemed to hang heavier than if it had been full, and it had echoes of ancient events repeated or time-locked, long ago.

We pulled up. Some nurses crunched over the gravel to collect me. There was some hesitation on the forecourt because I was scared of the moon. The situation just didn't seem *right*. My Mum said: "Don't you understand? *It's all happened before!"* And then I was back in, walking to my original room #102 as if along the last green mile from death row, back into the ward with doom hanging over me. This wasn't going to be the same experience I'd had in the place last time: no adventures.

I found plastic bags of clothes and belongings on my bed. The bags confused me. For a second I had believed they were mine but then a bearded, openly desperate, man came in and we stared at each other with a dawning horror: *"You're me!"* he said. *"I'm you!"* I replied. We were in the blackest trouble and both felt something akin to an acceptance of a 'cycle' without hope. I couldn't smoke and believed I'd come right 'off the rails'. I was given some tablets in the night-lighting outside the medication room and then the kind nurse, who had escorted me to my true room that night, had said as we'd passed a doorway to a dormitory of softly billowing curtains and snoring: "Try to be quiet – there are a lot of very old men in there." And I had thought that was nice. I also slept.

Three days later, mad for a cigarette or a cup of coffee, or both, I was escorted back to the Priory Hospital in Kent in a cab. This time I would be "there for the duration," as I've said sometimes, and during that first hospital 'set' (situation) I had fiddled about with pages of the *Nightbreed Chronicles* on a regular basis. I had given a page to the hospital priest, who had thanked me by name – even though we'd never met before – and I had stuck Boone and Lori's picture on the door of room #102. I had messed around with the book so much that when I was getting my shit together there was only one photograph left in the drawer. About to leave, in a state of severe withdrawal, I found the last page was a picture of the mad reverend *ASH*BURY.

On a Section Two of the Mental Health Act (1985) I arrived in Kent and was hustled into a room designed to the highest specification of entrapment at the bottom of the I C U. The plastic shower curtains had crisscrossing red and blue bars like Star Wars sabres. The bedspreads and curtains are woven into a greenish beehive of interlocking hexagons for that seized-up feeling. The door handles open upward so a patient can't open the door the usual way if they blunder to it in a blind panic. It's impossible to open the windows more than two inches because there is a black metal bar running tightly alongside them. The octagonal nursing station commands a view of both sides of the hospital with two metre edges. Hewn of quality wood, it has a complex telephone system under an over lapping top and is staffed 24 / 7. Needless to write there is a lot of medication about. Patients don't have to queue up for their foul pills and potions in this place, the prescriptions are brought to you in your room. No comfort.

On the first night I ran up the corridor and jumped over the Nurse's Station desk into the arms of a Pakistani doctor named Mammoud Mahendron. Since the apocalypse on the Island had failed to materialise everything was moving up a gear, the stakes were raised. The next setting would be England, and then it would be the world. On the third night in that place I really did 'flip out'. I wanted to get through the green automatic fire doors down at the bottom of the corridor and I was *scu*-driven to do this with *real fire*. After I put a few little things into a little bag such as contact lens stuff and a small picture of Kate, I placed a mixed pile of clothes in the middle of the floor, struck a match, and set it alight. The flames caught fast, licking tongues, alien and as hot as anger. Dense smoke funnelled into the room. The fire alarms were loud clanging bells, so loud, and I blanked out stumbling through the smoke but I got outside somehow. I felt like a back-seat passenger in my own head. Under cover of the darkness I walked across the car park past some firefighters who I saw shoving a metal pole through the window, perhaps to make an access hole for a hose, or to equalise the air-pressure, or something. I crossed the gravel, my shoes crunching unheard, and my old lungs filled with cool air like a soothing balm. Turning to the right I walked down the road like a ghost.

Not knowing for how long I had blanked out, when I got to the intersection at the bottom it happened again. I was transfixed by some graffiti on a road sign. I thought it was *Nightbreed* language and I stared at it as though I was continually on the verge of knowing its secrets, knowing something that didn't exist as I had done so many other times in those days. A staff car drew up and took me back to the ward where I was coshed. I remember only one short exchange I had with my consultant, Doctor Murray before getting greased horrendously with Chlorpromazine. *The 'Nightbreed Chronicles'* photographer is called *Murray Close*. I asked my Doctor if I could have a telephone in my room and she replied: "There are no telephones here, Richard, only shit." Then the horror treatment began.

Day after day, night after night, I took sick slurps of thick syrup and Procyclodine tablets for the side affects and Tomazapam jellies for night sedation, which have since been banned. Lying in the warm safety of my room I made comparisons to the wet cold of being on the run at 'the end' of days. I hoped Rachel and Reza would come crashing through the windows and rescue me, but they didn't show up... and days became weeks. Overhearing the nursing station I imagined that there was an experiment going on indicated by lunches and dinner orders, a sort of 'food apocalypse'.

I stumbled around in Murray's sanctioned delirium with my brain feeling like it was being soaked in battery acid. It was a state-of-the-art equivalent of 'Victorian treatment'. Awoken from deep sleep to take sleeping pills, I lay under a net blanket thinking I was dead. I was losing weight and desperate to smoke or have a cup of coffee, or a mug of tea, or any kind of sugar. I had given up *everything* because of the energy that could have burned out my anonymity, and the withdrawal was magnified into physical pain by *scu* 'Matter-Collectors'.

These things ate my chest flesh for lack of sustenance and it hurt but I still didn't smoke and that's why I knew Ashbury's character was a stubborn masochist. Even in gentler times 'Matter Collectors' had been known to get me up in the middle of the night for a chilled Coke.

The scent of cigarettes crept up beneath my door and set my brain on fire. At the little TV lounge area up at the top of the unit often sat a young Asian woman who smoked all the time. I thought she was a nicotine representative, not only that, but also somehow that she was actually *made* of the stuff: I hope I'm not a racist; I'm just reporting what I thought at that time. She asked me regularly if wanted to have a Benson & Hedges. And I said "No, no, no!" all the time. I was hallucinating weird glyphs evaporating into the walls, white on white cartouches of gibberish as one moment blended forever into the blind vortex. And then I was put under the invisibility of a telepathy blanket – must have been – while Barker himself told everyone he will "Take me out of the loop," and heal me. So the monster had me all to himself.

He tortured me beyond all 'sane' or 'reasonable' measures of combat in war. The shower and loo adjacent to Room #5, (my room since after the fire) became a terrible place. The fan in my loo was quiet but it sounded like alarm bells clanging or a fire-engine. This psychosis was Barker's TOILET horror. If I switched the fan off I had to sit in the darkness when I sometimes sensed the expression "smell yourself," and I would hallucinate travelling into blue tunnels, slipping along the insides of pipes and around bends like I was disappearing up my own arse. I hadn't even known there was a war going on. It had been like I was a dying squirrel in a barrel being poked with a stick. Occasionally, I inscribed bits and pieces of sad stuff into the pages of next year's diary and some of it had been too damn clever for me to have written alone in such a mind-warp, proof of his presence – I write such as: "Act or act" and: "Don't turn your heart into a spade."

When my parents visited, I sat between them feeling like a criminal between two police officers. I asked them to remember the expression "orbiting round the halls" and bring me some black & silver Halls menthol and Orbit chewing gum. But the things just sat untouched in my drawer for weeks because of my brainlessness and an environment like a lunatic pin ball machine. I was brought caffeine-free / sugar-free Coke but when it went flat it was just silly brown liquid. My head sometimes gyrated to the left and once my mother had had to spoon me my ham salad while I wept.

I finally submitted to severe carbohydrate / sugar withdrawal, and wrote in my journal: "ate a stick of Kit Kat and a strawberry!" which must have tasted quite beautifully. Around that time God rescued me in my sleep. I have no true memory of how it had it happened because the last vestiges of the dream may have been altered by the enemy in a rapid cover-up but I woke up thinking that I had 'cheated'. Whatever really happened I awoke happily the next morning for a hearty breakfast and a shave. Evil would not have wanted this. And if Evil had been *on my side* it would not have wanted me coshed so uselessly for so long either. God healed me *because* of the cosh. He rescued me. Most doctors would have called it a miracle recovery. And I accepted a B&H from the Asian girl. It tasted so fine, a relief at last in terms of my suddenly full blood supply. I was a bit 'stoned' and a *tiny* bit fearful perhaps, but I enjoyed it. Then I heard a voice – and I don't think God would have said something like this, either, particularly not while I was smoking. "The world is on your shoulders."

One of the last notable things that happened to me during that I C U experience was when I saw a music video on *Top of the Pops* of the #1 song *"Killer"* by Admaski. It was dark and beautiful and powerful and I cranked it up loud. The voice of a black man named Seal sounded as serious as if he were singing down the barrels of a shot-gun and the lyrics were empowered with a deep bass-line like the containment of violence behind bullet-proof glass. He sang: "It's the *loneliness* that's the killer," while his head rotated on a green background sparkling with bolts of lightning. It made my hair stand on end.

I was taken off the cosh and re-proscribed *Stelazine*. These were blue tablets with an 'S' on them like fruit sweets called 'Skittles' but no child should ever be allowed within hand's reach of anything like them. Days passed, and I ate, and relaxed. I drank cool 'build-up' milkshakes. The battery acid sensation started drying up because of the new drug. My brain began to feel like a crispy walnut but it *did* return to me a grasp of situations that I hadn't been capable of dealing with for weeks. It was a 'dry' sensation but *much* more preferable to that initial shit storm of Chlorpromazine. I was becoming curious about therapy and asked about what groups and classes were going on 'out there'. One morning I was allowed to join a group actually *outside!!* Two days before I moved into the new atmosphere of the unsecured areas of the hospital I was put on the Early Morning Walk. I waited at a door in the corridor parallel to the restaurant with other people, *volunteer* patients that I had never met before, and I knew that shortly I would be seeing the colour blue above me instead of plaster, and green all around instead of painted walls. Not thought so clinically, it was more of an emotional anticipation of how amazing it was really going to be.

Whatever the professional's opinion about escape undercover of arson some might have said I had been locked up for too long. *I hadn't seen the sky for eleven and a half weeks.* Even if it hadn't really been quite this long, let's say nine weeks – it could still have been considered a breech of my human rights that never should have happened. We were actually going to walk *outside*. At 9AM two friendly Occupational Therapy staff arrived to friendly comments, cliquey "Good Mornings," and "Hellos," by name. The door was opened and we crossed the road into the cool morning sunlight. The birds were singing. We went into the woods, a place of light like the tide in a tropical sea. The air of the forest was continuously energising, pushing the desire to continue like the trees were leading an aerobics class. The trees themselves were many shades of green with crusty velvet trunks that climbed up and up like the tallest living things I had ever seen. And, above even those, was a blue sky: so huge, so up, away, and so big, it seemed impossible that we didn't all just fall off the world.

I went walking most mornings but several weeks later I started sliding back to some of my old ways. Maybe it was the essences of mental recovery, like sleeping in for many extra hours until lunch, yet it was a happy time and I felt a genuine optimism. I shared it like laughter with some new friends. Salley-faye (her entire head braded with coloured beads): old man Peter (owner & director of an Audio Visual firm in Shepherds Bush): and drinking endless cups of filter coffee with Justin (who wouldn't have said "boo" to a goose but who had nevertheless told me he had broken through the wall into his neighbour's living room with a sledge hammer) and I was 'doing': good, happy, things.

Another brilliance, there was the friendship I built with Peter. We 'talked shop', about creativity, and I showed him a collection of some of the best photographs I had ever taken that Peter said could have been shot by a professional! I told him about the forthcoming cinema release of *Nightbreed* in some detail and he suggested that maybe I shouldn't watch it. One day his new Production Director came down from the capitol and I must have made a good impression on both men because they offered me a job! *At last I had a foot in the door* and it explained, to some extent, the reason *why* I had gone through all of this shit. I was to start working in 1991 as a Junior Production Assistant in London!

By August I was 'back to sleep'. The horror impossibilities of fate and my terrifying psychosis had gone. It didn't seem so bad to return to a bit of hashish because I believed, then, that my being 'well' meant being how I had been *before all this crazy stuff had happened*. I smoked it even though I was still on the ward and it made my brain feel like shit. I did it perhaps to prove my newfound freedom, inadvertently casting some dark seeds to the four winds. They would originate weeds that would drag me down choking later into some new madness.

CHAPTER FIVE: *1991 / Hospital Two*

I began writing in 1988 and the work was a mishmash of role models from which my own style would emerge. I wrote to repair the ego destruction of grilling meat. By that summer in Hayse Grove I had only reached 132 pages of my book but I knew somehow that I would finish it. The name of Peter's new Director of Production was Max and I had heard he spoke Arabic and Hebrew fluently. He was a tall, calm man with long sandy hair in a ponytail, his eyes sharp and blue. The vitality of the meeting was lost to me yet Peter let me know that the job was mine if I wanted it.

Months passed. I bought a 'step-through' Honda moped. I was passionate when discussing "being well" with my parents but I was taking drugs again. I smoked a little hashish with Tony Hill but we no longer had anything in common. In the spring of 1991 when freezing weather was powdering the roads and gardens of the Island, my old friends and I took a tab of L.S.D each for a "trip through the snow". It would be the last I would take because of one of the maddest most terrible sensations I have ever felt.

An ancient constituent in the recipe for L.S.D is 'strychnine', a deadly muscular poison in larger quantities. I don't know whether it was this chemical that had caused the trouble or if it was some other component but the very method of escape – going to sleep – had itself been triggering the nasty reaction. A sub-thought came to me that it was a "marple": as I slipped into shallow sleep I felt deep, hideous acidic stuff being squeezed off in the very centre of my brain. So, I would jump awake, and I couldn't get away from it. I rolled around, groaning, while every so often my pituitary gland would again spasm. I don't think *Scu* had been involved, or "attack raptures" yet it was a chemical reaction so shitty I have never taken the stuff since, nor will again. I have a delicate brain.

On the train to London I listened to Seal's first album, and *"Blissed Out"* by Beloved; Orbital, and sometimes *"Real Life"* by Simple Minds. I had a bookshelf in my room but I didn't read often. On that shelf was a book Ellie had given me as research for *'Necronomicon'* called the *Book of Black Magic*. I didn't read that either. I ate a lot during the months following the hospital. A psychologist might have said that it was because I was afraid my food was going to be taken away. At other times I felt so exhausted after eating I needed to sleep so I went to 'rest', rationalised it as being a result of digestion – although it had been barely eight o'clock in the evening. Their assault had been exerted out of malicious sadism. I was oblivious to thousands of similar attacks. I knew of no war.

I saw Barker's movie *"Nightbreed"* three times. He had written, produced and directed a remarkable vision of the *Cabal* prophesy. The creatures his cast brought to life had essences of something that I had needed for a long time, a family that could understand and forgive. I bought a 'T' shirt with Boone on the front in his monstrous state, and I received a couple of letters from Max. They were always a small pleasure. Near my 22nd birthday while the biting chill of winter was thawing I found a bed-sit in London, in Hammersmith. It was a top floor square room with its own fridge and a shared kitchen downstairs. The bed seemed comfortable enough to sleep on. I liked it. It was a short walk from Goldhawk Road station and not too many minutes further to get to work in a cul-de-sac in Shepherds Bush. My father drove my possessions and myself to the house in late March and helped me set up my home. About six days later I started work.

It began on a grey Monday morning, cold outside my duvet, but I dressed quickly. I cooked a breakfast of tinned tomatoes and mushrooms on toast and then started walking with a jaunty step. My enthusiasm was the bow of an ice-breaking ship in the arctic. The front door was locked because I had been so keen I had arrived 45 minutes early! I probably felt that I waited by that red front door longer than I really did. About half an hour later a pretty woman in black clothes walked up the steps. She introduced herself as

Penny, Max's secretary, and she unlocked the door. We went inside. I had my little notebook ready.

I was excited and maybe a little anxious to have been accepted into this clique. They were interesting people who perhaps couldn't remember being a new face themselves, their own versions of what I was feeling then. I saw some fantastic tools like a huge 64 channel audio mixer, and being at last on the *inside* was making me a man of responsibility. My usual work was to deliver or collect packages from other firms around London, which was how I became exposed to a city that does not stop. The sights and sounds and smells batter you continuously – the fumes of jammed traffic, of cars and bikes rumbling everywhere. The strangers on the clogged streets who never look at the sky, highly strung people who have the same pitch of consciousness like everyone is constantly on the same lane of motorway. And the advertising is like a hurricane... a loud storm of *marketing* on such an utterly huge scale it defies acknowledgement. It flows past the eyes like newspaper pages unspooling in a grey blur from a press, not glossed over but unprocessed – and if you did take it in you'd have a problem. It was good to get back to my parents at the weekends where I sometimes went dancing.

There was a war going on in the Gulf. Surreal images of the night sky over Israel lit with the tail fires of missiles made green and futuristic through the light sensitive film-stock. Troop gatherings, tanks blatting their guns at each other in the desert, and Kate Adie reporting defiantly from the front line. After three weeks my job became more difficult. I began to re-experience poisoned thoughts but I felt good. My pituitary gland was producing extra endorphins. I felt strong.

When I took out a Marlboro I sometimes uttered a dope reference: "Let's get a number together..." Radiating power again, I thought that I was a kind of 'battery' for the firm and that this guaranteed my position. But there's more to a job than smoking cigarettes and drinking coffee. I was losing concentration, I was losing grip. My whereabouts were known and I felt I was like a 'baby god'. I pinned a couple of bizarre poems to the staff notice board and I was getting messages from people, subliminal and secretive. 'Co-incidences' came by the dozen and I called it 'K' input – synchronicity from above like traffic signals changing to WALK when it was required, flicking randomly through paper-backs to uncover coherent sentences. And attention grabbing to posters upon was written such as "Children should be seen and not hurt" and "We believe in life before death". I dressed in hippy clothes from Carnaby Street on a mental plateau, but I had no firm friends to talk to so I expressed myself at home via a collage.

I tacked pictures to the walls of my room; album covers, observations of light and dark, of Art conspiracy and telepathy. The wall beside my door was a learning curve in itself, a 'third effect' of frozen movement that by the end of my time in London had numbered over 50 pictures. Some of these expressed my loneliness and my need of a lovely girlfriend. Interior *sub-thought* pointed out that the *Nightbreed* wanted me to have a girlfriend also – a chip off my spiritual mother's old block. The Earth originator of her group is the respected and mysterious Kate. I felt a strong connection with her when I heard her #1 hit *"Wuthering Heights"* and I sometimes found myself pausing if I snatched the song played on radio or television. I got a ring given to me by my flesh mother Liz and I wore it like a mooring rope securing the safety of a yacht. But when it actually came to finding a girlfriend the art of seduction was an enigma to me. I was as inept as the next lonely man in the city.

On the first bank holiday in May I left work quickly with a suitcase too fat for three days. There was to be dancing all night on Sunday and I was anticipating an added enjoyment through the exercise of anonymous power. I rode the Central Line wearing hippy cotton trousers of yellow and ochre patchwork, the *Boone* merchandise 'T' shirt with the sleeves cut off, and a Hawaiian shirt of colourful Paisley draped over my shoulders. The train pulled into a station and then something happened that has never been repeated since in the same way. I had a meeting with the *Nightbreed*, face to face, and it was the last thing I would have expected.

A blonde 30-something woman sat opposite me and plonked her string tied shoulder bag between her thighs. She looked at me in a frank appraisal. She carried on looking at me. So I said: "see anything you like?" which had taken surprisingly little courage. / "That 'T' shirt," she replied: "I know someone who was in that film." / "Oh yes?" / "Who was the creature with snakes in his hair?" she asked. And of course I knew this. I said "Peloquin!" Then, a new question began to hover in the air in rattling carriage between us, an invitation... but I didn't want to meet the man who had played that creature. Riding my inflated mass ego-powered rocket of pride I nevertheless indicated my suitcase and told her I was going home. She looked a bit disgusted, which had seemed appropriate somehow. Then she said: "I'm his wife!" and got off the train at the next stop.

I believed I could have gone with her. Maybe the chance had been there. But I had experienced a thought afterwards, of dubious origins, that my cowardice may have saved my life. If 'they' were blaming my energy for aggravating the Gulf War I might have followed Peloquin's wife to my grave. There were soberer explanations, of course, those 'black miracles' randomly worsening illness by verifying psychotic belief. Back on the Island my mum Liz heard what had happened and she dismissed the event with a similar sobriety.

Becoming re-concerned about my Marlboro habit I shook a twenty-sided dice before going out that weekend and allowed it to choose how many I could smoke at the 'rave'. There were two All-Nighters being held: at *"Too Too's"*, on the road to Clacton, and in the Hippodrome on Colchester High Street. The answer to where I would go popped up when I was reading a sliding text sign in a restaurant – an expression something like **"2 for the price of 2"** – and that decided it. I was physically sick over a cigarette with excitement and excess endorphins on the way. The dice had allocated me eleven cigarettes, and, to use modern console-gaming language, they were 'power-ups'.

"Too Too's" was kicking that night, with heat, music, and lighting. Sweating dancers passing around bottles of mineral water, movements stuttering in the strobe light... I danced on a platform to the thunder of an apocalyptic bass like the rapid launches of self-propelled rockets. The laser guided speckled shards of light in intentional lines and patterns that blended with the music into a manifestation of awesome power. I had a hugely over-inflated opinion of myself. I was enjoying the blackest of global possibilities and called this dance "The Armageddon Rave". I concluded after attention grabs to purple lights that they represented 'ultra chaos'. I never knew what it actually meant – just that it was potent and at this time such potency was mine. My 'superiority complex' evolved into the ego of a mad deity as I lorded it over the others around me from the platform. I was a master and they were going to hell for stealing from heaven. Being in a nightclub is fun, but not if you're stuck in one forever. I sometimes called such places MAX, colloquial for certain prisons.

With about two songs to go by my watch I found half a cigarette on the edge of the stage as though it had been placed there especially, and it tasted fine, a rush to fill up depleted energy levels. Then I saw the reflection of an EXIT sign in the mirrors and took my leave, walked straight out to find a taxi that wasn't booked outside. I took it comfortably back to Mersea while *Radio One* played a song called *"See the Lights"* by Simple Minds – *which I had seen.* It was from an album called *"Real Life"* that had threads of prophesy through it. The last track is called *"When Two Worlds Collide..."* Following that the station played *"I Can't Get No*

Satisfaction" by the Rolling Stones... and I figured that was fair sarcasm.

In my parents' garden early that morning I studied a flyer advertising the next rave: a silhouette of a figure with outstretched arms against a background of perhaps Chaos: the patterns of repetition within repetition called Mandlebroth Sets. The dance was entitled "CHANGES" and I considered it a suitable name for a future event. But I was never to see it. Soon, from the height of my elevated sense of self, I was going to crash down hard from an oblivious sky.

By Tuesday I was back at work, smoking nicotine-free cigarettes that I had bought from a pharmacy called "Honey Rose". They smelt like cannabis although I had sworn myself off that also, but this alternative cigarette wasn't going to be enough. I had been accustomed to an unnaturally high quota of bliss brain chemicals for too long, an exaggeration of the glands that produced endorphins. In plain language the alteration had been an attack or, as Barker's manipulations have since become known to me, it was*"Rapture"*. Logic dictates that they used few matter-collectors because they wouldn't have wanted me to start smoking Marlboro again. They just wanted me to be in a compromising position and it couldn't have happened in a worse place than London.

The following Saturday I started talking to a neighbour in the kitchen in Hammersmith, a woman who had been raised in Denmark aged about twenty-five. Sexually speaking she wasn't really my type but "beggars can't choose" was not the way I accepted women, it wasn't an aspect of my masculinity. She told me there was a rock concert going on in Finsbury Park that night featuring: *Killing Joke, New Model Army,* and ending with *The Mission,* which was a band I particularly liked. It sounded like a fantastic line-up so we went together. A tout outside sold us cheap tickets I doubted were authentic enough to get us in but I needn't have worried. We got in with no difficulty. Traders skirted the edge of the field and lots of young people in dark 'alternative clothing' were milling about. A few could be seen dancing to the first band, and others were sitting about in groups drinking, and smoking, and chatting. I surveyed this arena from the back of the field. It was as though I was looking into a dome containing exotic fish that I couldn't touch. However, I knew I needed a partner and since there were plenty of fish in these waters I left the Danish woman. I said I would "catch up with her later", and got into a little boat called hope.

On the left of the field I sat down next to a brunette and dredged up an opening line. She was well spoken with blue eyes, and she was wearing small boots and a dress of dark velvet. We talked. She was over twenty and worked as a graphic designer and I figured my own job as a junior production assistant was comparable. She was pretty and that aggravated my natural fear of failure and the added unnatural fear generated by *scu*. This girl was a beautiful parcel that I felt too afraid to open because there was an epiphany within it, a possibility that this night could be amazing, that I might end up with this girl on my arm at the front of a crowd to a band whose name I would have considered apt – *The Mission*. It was possible that it could be the next night of the rest of my life but I couldn't talk to her. I had found her in the sea using my boat but the wind had dropped and my sails were useless. Good things can cause fear as well as bad sometimes. There were *push-sub-thoughts* of a cusp in destiny that I couldn't cope with so I told her I would meet her by the 'burger bus' at half past eleven, and then pulled the plug. I never saw her again.

I wandered aimlessly in a *scu*-created mental annexe. I bought an ice-cream and a bottle of Irish carbonated mineral water from some traders. I was made to feel as though I was 'welshing' and displayed the cone to attentive telepaths as though I was yearning for childhood. I dribbled white spills onto my jeans, a spectacle many would have considered sexual. It didn't enter my mind that I could no longer be a child and that I wasn't allowed to get through it that way. I was a man having a cop-out and retired from the area understanding I might not have been able to plug back into that crowd even if I'd wanted to. I left Finsbury Park like a whipped dog with the Irish water bottle under my arm like the dog's plastic bone. I wobbled directionless through the streets having diseased adventures even though I didn't hear 'voices' in those days.

Immersed in empathy rather than telepathy I began 'Caballing' my spiritual family. They were the forces of nature and I balanced them, then, *six years* before I would become a full 'receiver' in 1997. Flashes rippled through my brain connecting my thoughts like knuckles of forked lightning. I concluded purple Amethyst was a mother's stone and that the Irish water-force's stone was Opal since Katherine had given me a small jarful. Rejecting Kate in favour of the West I pulled off the ring my mum had given me and I threw it against a wall. Sensing more adventures to be had in this senseless rambling, I went looking for them. To this day I don't remember how I got back home to Hammersmith. Could have been on the Tube, or a taxi? It wouldn't have been a bus (I rarely took them); maybe I walked? Whatever, when I was back I needed comfort.

I went to the room of the Danish woman and asked her for a cuddle, nothing more, and she allowed me under her duvet. My middle name is Mark and I felt her platonic companionship be the allocation of a safe house – a den – because of her country *Denmark*. We watched TV and I felt my adventures had become common knowledge to the Artists because there was a war film being shown on the BBC that was, unavoidably, "A Bridge Too Far." They were trying to tell me something but I was bone tired and wanted it all to stop. The *scu* scared me out of her bed. I went back to my own where I could forget. I fell asleep. It was so deep I couldn't see the bars of psychosis strengthening the cage around me.

My first pay-cheque was amazing, like finding a gold ticket to visit the Wonk Chocolate Factory! Max wanted me to sort his filing cabinet but I had no idea how it could be done. I figured he was testing me. Like a storm blowing my windmill the task was a gale rotating the fan so hard it was threatening to tear the sails off. I would like to write I was happy. I would like to write I was blasé, and could cope with anything, but those days were ebbing away. I had been working at the firm only four weeks but the job had become so difficult I needed a few days off. Max gave me until the following Wednesday, and so I made arrangements to visit a couple of my parents' friends in Wiltshire, David and Sal, for a break.

I think it may have been the Friday evening that I got on the train. The couple lived in a converted mill with lots of cats and dogs, well-read, gentle people. I had thought they were my friends also but you might agree perception is all and I couldn't sense my love returned. They were supposed to meet me off the train at Hungerford but I had got as far as Reading carrying my typically distended suit-case. I used my imagination to project images of a different locale in case I was being followed. I don't recall having enough cash left on me for even a phone call so in the waiting area I asked a young man for spare change and he seemed to give me all the money he had, which was odd. I called David and Sal and soon they picked me up and drove us into the dark countryside.

Their initial smiles and hugs were tarnished by my illness. I couldn't connect with them. Their home was a honey-trap, a different world to my own. It was a place of dog-eared carpets and wood and interesting books. They sponged information off me and I detected a unit of supernatural minds. I began to think their place was a taster of some kind of After-life – yet I didn't want to see it. However beautiful the mill, it was too early to consider my 'retirement', too early to think about dying. When I choked on points of discussion they tried to reel me in, kindly, but I already had the answer to my assessment. They were prison officers from Hell and that night I went to bed knowing that I had to get out as soon as I could.

On the following morning, Saturday, I did. I hefted my heavy case down the drive, exerting myself towards a train station with no knowledge of where it was. It may have been several miles away so what you might have expected to happen next, did: David picked me up in his car. He drove me to a cash-point and saw me on my way back to London. By this juncture I was so far out of my gourd I was soon to be push-subbed around again like the robot I had been the year before. I was being shunted along a doomed destiny line on another train. The tracks were all going down. "Welcome to the Night Train," you might have said. "The next stop is Hell on earth".

On Sunday night I got it into my head to go somewhere else. I was going to walk from London to Cornwall – reading meanings in nothing. So you can understand this common distortion of schizophrenia here are two examples: that I would rub my feet with sores, walking all the way to 'Corn – wall', on a 'bridge' with no turning back – the *Uxbridge Road* – where other rabid adventures took place. I believed the comic Billy Connolly was doing a show at the time, on a live link to me while I was walking; 'in-jokes' about the randomness of this crazy lord. I paced a long way and found some long plastic pipes stacked near a sign that said the road-works would be completed in 1992. I was too early! Walking back the way I had come in the small hours of Monday morning I hitched a lift with a man in a green car. After he had dropped me off it seemed that he was followed by someone else in a red car but there was nothing I could do about telepaths playing 'car wars'. The sun was to rise soon. I decided I would go back to work, return two days before the arrangement I'd struck with Max. If I thought I was feeling happy and breezy that morning, that I would 'be on the ball' at the office, I was delusional. I had had no sleep.

Sorting my boss's files was the final scrambling aspect of a scrambled mind, like a weight so heavy it wasn't worth *even trying* to lift it. In the afternoon I stood in a bright storage room downstairs barely comprehending I was holding a pair of stainless-steel scissors in my right hand. I wasn't suicidal; I just needed to cut myself awake. I pressed the point of a blade into my other hand, the only tiny movement in a mindless seizure. I made a tiny cut and a little blood welled up... then I crashed out of that brain-lock into a terrible new world. No one could have imagined what I was going through. Even if some of the telepaths upstairs actually *did* know, they could not have interfered in the Material 'vicinity' without blurting crazy stuff out loud. A part of me *did* blame them for it. I should have got through the whole thing without one single drop of blood. Wherever I went, whatever I did, through the riots, hell, or high water, I was supposed to reach the last moment without even a scratch. And yet here was blood and even because of a very tiny cut, the situation was going to the wall *and I had shed it myself.*

On the Tuesday morning my plateau fell through the floor. I was told Max wanted to see me. I must have known what was coming but I couldn't take it in initially. Max started with "We are going to have to let you go." I may have felt like I was watching myself on a screen yet the metaphor falls through itself because of how lifeless I felt compared to the high emotions, paradoxically, of a movie. So I just said: "OK," then most likely: "I'm sorry." This was reality. Max said: "You want glory, Richard, and there is no glory to be had in this job." / "Do you want me clear out my desk?" / "No.

We'll post it to you... just go." So, for the last time, I walked out of the office. I advanced into the mania of London where my adventuring was shifting from harmless theory into deadly reality.

I found a Job Agency and went inside. I was briefly interviewed. The agent, a hard-bitten woman, told me that if I was lucky I might be able to get a job grilling burgers. Reality crashed in on me again as I walked out. I had fallen from the best job in the world to the opportunity of only the shittiest recollection of Bristol, and maybe I had also lost my 'mask'; I had no professional status by which people are judged. No 'umbrella' to protect me from the dangers of the capitol. I walked on with that strange but familiar randomness, and walked, and walked… and then found myself outside BBC Television Centre. So here it was. I had found the shop-floor of perhaps the tightest clique on Earth, that like many others I idolised. I went into the glass security office.

A guard said that I couldn't talk to anyone without an appointment. Even if I had made a proper arrangement, with the likes of Personnel, my C.V was looking unmentionable. The guard gave a contact number that I lost quickly. I stood by the gates, brain-locked again, and then distantly absorbed the fact that the bar was being raised for a car. I saw a light turn from red into green – and then I suddenly snapped. I ducked under the opening and walked up the right hand side of the road without looking back. I was as tense as if spirits with sniper rifles were suspended behind me but I was outwardly calm. Inside a part of me expected a shout or a raised hand to bring me trouble that I could neither imagine nor need.

Treading over wood chippings, the kind you might find on a children's playground, I walked past a disused fountain in an area enclosed on three sides with glass walls. I pushed onto the door ahead of me. It opened and inside I found a sign on the wall discussing three possible fire-escape routes (coloured red, blue and green) and I went upstairs. The 2nd level was composed underfoot of black tiles, maybe an acoustic floor, and along the wall were numbered doors. I knocked on #5, which was probably a *push-sub-thought* of the Enemy because five is the '*caballing* number' – the centre of four – and a voice said: "Come in!"

Inside there was a grey-haired gentleman I didn't recognize, but who asked: "How did you know where to find me?!" And I thought that was a really *great* reaction so I got right down to the problem I was having: "I've been sacked from an audio-visual firm in Shepherds Bush. Do you anyone I can talk to about getting a job?" So he said: "Wait here. I'll just go get a friend of mine..." The door *was not* crashed through by a gang of stampeding heavy weight security men. Instead the man returned with his friend just like he had said he would do. Except that this friend was a tall man, with cropped hair and eyes of blue steel who looked more like a policeman than do most policemen. I told them: "I think we'll use the Blue Route..." but in all honesty this was a scrap of crap I'd gleaned off the fire-escape notice board. The tall man said: "We can't help you, *we're only actors.*"

Not really understanding this I asked him what I should do. He positively radiated the Law, and he said: "Go to 46 Marshall Street." My doctor back home was called Dr. Marshall. / "What's there?" "The Samaritans..." Then Security did arrive. The tall man instructed them to just take me out – as if telling them simultaneously not to rough me up, or anything – and there were at least five, all asking at once about how I'd gained access to the building, but the Q & A was kind of hazy. Then I was back on the street. The sun was going down on my last day of freedom in London.

After another 'ice-cream cop-out', outside the tube-station on Shepherds Bush Green I walked back to Hammersmith. I never did get to Marshall Street. When I was talking to the bloke in the ice cream van ("How much do you want it to cost?" he'd asked me!) I had thought he was a telepath too, another one pissed off by my inept behaviour regarding the collapsing Boone prophesy. Back at 'home' my room was like an icebox, with an open window that I don't recall closing. It was as cold as the cockpit of a yacht in the arctic with rogue winds pushing the boat near lethal icebergs. And I felt that my time was going; just *going*...

I put the TV on and I heard an announcer say: "There will be a special surprise for you at eight o'clock." I set my watch alarm for that time and in mathematics the figure eight lying on its side represents Infinity. I switched off the set and bumbled around the room. I didn't notice that a Kate Bush album lay beside the Irish mineral water next to my dusty word processor. I didn't *want to* notice because it was sad – I hadn't opened the bottle, nor listened to the disc for weeks or typed a single word into the computer since before I arrived.

Grains of sand were pouring away. There is a bubble on each end of an hour-glass; it doesn't care either way. I was being led out to a chopping block and I didn't need to tell the time to understand it was running out. An attention grab led my eyes to my book-shelf and I walked up to it reaching for something… a paperback with a distant greyness… it was *The Book of black Magic*… I picked it up and opened it as my alarm suddenly and LOUDLY BEEPED the 'infinity hour'… an ink diagram of a conjuration sampled from ancient grimours – a stylised boat adorned with odd markings - ancient symbols, and I read the title of the curse and I was thunderstruck. It was the *"SEAL OF BUNE"*.

Scu shoved a spanner into my 'word-to-audio converter' because the explanation I read was altered. I found out what had *actually* been written later. What I had believed then, in that moment alone in that room at the hour of infinity, was that the *Seal of Bune* had taken my spirit and left me as an empty shell. It had 'raptured' my soul into a brother who had been still born, long ago, and now this sibling had a soul. He could be born again and I was rendered hollow at a fundamental level. This curse had taken my soul and soon it would be time for me to take the life.

Like someone stoned on dope having cold water chucked in his face I stumbled away from the bookshelf and swayed in the middle of the room looking at the table. The title of the Kate Bush C.D was *"NEVER FOREVER"*. I took a step toward the Irish mineral water and at a distance of three feet the bottle suddenly *hissssed* at me like a snake, an outburst from an unbroken cap. My options were being destroyed. Nobody may ever adequately explain these events yet they nonetheless happened. My mind pondered. When I felt the situation could be better outside I walked downstairs. I was thinking slowly yet an express train was underway. Things were going fast. It was cold here on the streets, also, but there was no relaxation in the black 'K' perception. I found a clock in a window divided into four colours indicating a quarter to nine. The clock was behind bars, and near the expression "*TIME OUT*". I went back upstairs.

The chance that death might cause me to cease to exist, *nullify*, had been concealed. It didn't occur to me then because I felt I had no option, that death was necessary after my material and spiritual redundancy. Whatever strange thing I had been here to do, I had utterly failed and it was time to leave the game. Even faster now, trying to slow things down, I ate half a bar of Hayse Grove hospital soap over the sink. With my mouth stinging with sick and soap burns I had thoughts like that death was 'honourable' and 'brave'. I thought Gillette razors were "The Mark of a Man" so I sat on the edge of my bed cutting myself with a broken disposable razor and a blunt bread knife...

I gave up half an hour later. I used a clean yellow duster and strapped it tight over my gash with tape, then sedated my mouth ulcers with a long draft of the fizzy Irish water. It was cream soda, cool and beautiful as ice vanilla. The current run of failure had to be applied to suicide as well as to every thing else. I couldn't even do *that* properly, so I decided I would leave. Just get dressed into warm clothes and leave. I packed my camera bag with some basic toiletries, my blue pillow case, wallet, possibly my Walkman, and a small photo of my parents (bitter irony?) – and, of course, my SLR camera – then pulled on a brown leather jacket and left the door open so anyone could take whatever they wanted. I never saw that room again.

I stepped outside onto the pavement like I was poking a stick at something I couldn't see clearly. I decided I would be a street level photographer, which was a dangerous occupation; there were thoughts that I hadn't got the balls for it even after what I had done to myself... but if I had the courage, what had I got to lose? The answer was that I had my *freedom* to lose. I started walking and my characteristic randomness straightened out. I followed *pushed-sub-thoughts*. I wouldn't be hearing 'voices' for another five and a half years but this was the <u>loudest silence</u> I had ever experienced! Empathy like non-visual memory guided me 'left / right / straight on' and I felt myself being led towards the safe house of the *Nightbreed*. I found a red door marked #1, opposite a van marked "Carpets and Furniture" and I thought of *Weaveworld*. Somewhere else a chequered flag marked journey's end.

I rang the bell. There was no answer. A thought suggested I must prove myself to them by throwing my camera through the basement window. If I *did throw it* they would finally welcome me in... I decided to do it. I unscrewed the lens and tightened a body-cap onto the camera, then flung it into the room that was to the bottom left of the front door, a basement room window behind a set of black bars a few feet 'roadside of the window' thus *not protected* by the railing. The camera wasn't in my hands anymore. There were screams from inside after a loud BANG of glass and I climbed down over the railings and started smashing at the hole with my right shoe. I sussed what had happened. I had broken the Law as irreparably as I had broken the window. And as I looked back at the van some of the letters of the sign 'Carpets & Furniture' were obscured. I climbed onto the bed, then onto the floor, stunned into a total brain-lock by what I read through the railings. The expression: "AR PET".

It felt like I had been standing there for barely thirty seconds but I must have been 'out' for at least eight minutes. Before I realized the crime and the likely termination of my freedom, that I had been crushed yet again by mental illness, there were uniform police officers all over me. They dragged me through the house into the back of a van, and drove it to Shepherds Bush police station. I remember there were several officers hanging about while the desk sergeant went through my property as if they had nothing better to do. There were jokes about the 'Life Boy' soap, and other sarcasm I didn't understand. I stood there desperate for a cigarette while other people were smoking so I asked if my pillow case could be sealed in an evidence bag before its delicate scent could be ruined. The police surgeon arrived. He examined my wrist then taped it up with two 'butterfly' stitches and asked if I wanted a sleeping tablet. Like a bloody idiot I said "No" and was locked in a cell.

It was like being inside a disused chamber-pot stored in a place no one had looked into for months. There was a toilet hidden in alcove, tiling the colour of old crockery, and a bare tungsten bulb hanging from the ceiling. Out of reach. In my pockets I found a small piece of opal, a pair of socks, and a Biro. There was an unbreakable window of thick opaque squares of safety glass that seemed dirty. Because of the continuous lighting there could be no shadows but for my own, of course, which was rapidly becoming all that was left of me.

I slung my leather jacket onto the 'bed', a bench covered in torn red vinyl, then stood under the window with a piece of opal gripped in the thumb and forefinger of my right hand. I cracked it and suddenly the force, which I had been thinking of it as *"The Art",* flew through the safety glass in a gusher of symbols like water through a broken dam. This was energy produced by my daily functions and somehow stored in another 'vicinity' within me. In my fear of its affect I had even air-attacked it from myself, because it warped people, but at this moment the passing of these weird shapes and glyphs was a cusp between abandonment and the need to carry on being 'important'. So I re-gripped the shards of opal and it stopped the fire works. I'd lost about 60% of the total.

I hallucinated horrid little beetles scuttling about on the floor and I tried to suffocate myself on my leather jacket, which felt as though I was crinkling up in a madness of shrinking smaller and when I reached the size of a bean I gave up… then I set to attacking my left wrist again with the Biro but the wound hurt too much. So I worked on the other, instead. Then I had to cover up what had happened – soaked up the damage with the socks and put them behind the toilet. Perhaps after that I may have slept, but that night I was never given a blanket, or a rug, and all I got for breakfast was a paper cup of tea and a biscuit.

A few minutes after drinking the tea I was wondering if I could use the energy it produced to 'chip myself out of the sandbox' when Social Services arrived. The door had been unlocked and in walked a heavy-set man with short blonde hair. I went eye to eye with him. He was a social worker, and he had his own assessment to do. When he began questioning me I realised that he was Irish and that he had almost total power over my future. My answers were psychotic; the act of a healthy mind concealing illness, but I couldn't win because the damaged wrists were the only proof he really needed to apply the Mental Health Act. He talked me into having my injuries dressed at Charing Cross Hospital and said that's all we would do, but he had lied... If I hadn't been talked into going onto the psychiatric wards I would have been dragged up to them kicking and yelling anyway.

My trauma was eased by a pretty nurse. She used warm water and I felt a comforting relief at her touch and the clean tightness of her bandaging. Then I walked through a side door onto the street. A thought came to me then that I should *run for it* but there was no substance to the idea. I didn't want to. The Irishman appeared through another side door about 14 feet down, came up the road, and led me indoors to his office. When he was sitting at his desk he asked me for my parent's telephone number. He began dialling my Dad, far away, in Mersea, and a great tide of regret welled up inside me, the final deep knowledge that I had gone to the city with such great hopes and all had crashed to nothing. So I cried... and a thought came to me then that a man with no soul wouldn't be able to. Maybe I had recovered something. Maybe I was to be incarcerated more 'together' than since leaving work yesterday.

We went up in a lift and got off on the 7th Floor. He began to lead me towards the East Ward and I could see through the glass essences in there of fresh air and pictures and flowers. Yet I balked, tried to pull away, weakly, thinking that I was acting out what I was supposed to do. So the social worker said: "Well, if that's how you want it," and pulled me into the West Ward. There were sheets of wire reinforced glass everywhere with seven rooms marked 'A' to 'G', including a bath that looked more like an instrument of torture. It was a hell-hole of hard nurses with strong medication and passive smoke that would set my brain on fire. The Irishman released me. I wandered down the corridor and found a punk in room 'A' who asked me what I was doing there. I told him I was the Anti-Christ. He said: "welcome home."

I would have treated myself with more kindness if I could have just got out of there, back into the East Ward, but I was a poisoned mouse looking for an antidote in a maze. I was under OBS '1' – close nursing supervision. The scu were driving me around and there was no escape. The nurses' behaviour drove me also and the combination had me looking for an end to it. I hadn't been eating much fruit or roughage for a long time and while on a loo in a room that most would have seen as worse than my cell in Shepherds Bush station, while straining away the light bulb blew. I was suddenly plunged into darkness and the nurse that looked round the door at me said: "Look what you've done now!" After being driven to play with my crap I washed and wandered off. At the back of the nurses station I found a store-room and dismissed the brief thought of drinking bleach. Instead, I tried to fall onto the Biro as I had once read in a book – about a knife – at angle up under the rib cage into my heart – but the torn skin hurt badly, so I gave that a miss as well.

Back in my room there was a big sheet of plywood obscuring the night-time view surrounding the hospital. A nurse just inside the door saw me lying in bed with a pyjama top tied around my neck. I was trying to asphyxiate myself and he said something like: "I'll give you five minutes to do it." Or perhaps said: "I'll come back in five minutes and see if you've done it," or something equally horrid. Morning was coming... I started looking at the rectangle of plywood covering the window as the dim light brightened around it. I suspected it was a replacement for the inside pane of the double glazing. I thought about Migs, recalled him telling me: "You've got to try a bunji-jump, Rich. You get so much adrenaline you'll be buzzing for a week after!" I thought about this and saw the wood adhered to the frame with tiny 'tack' nails. I thought about it a lot. There was a chair beneath the hole. The missing window was usually made of glass so toughened it probably verged bullet-proof, but the outside pane was weak. And then I knew I was going to jump.

At about half past six I went to the nursing station and asked for a cup of tea and a newspaper. A push-sub-thought made me believe Boone had requested such in 'connected circumstances', in the prophesy but Boone never jumped out of a window in *'Cabal'*. I sat on the chair, my heart beating fast. The news headlines scuttled past my eyes like invisible rodents. I sipped the tea, my heart beating quicker. It was a grey day outside, the light brighter now. I dropped the empty paper cup and the empty paper of news on the bed, and placed the chair under the window. My heart was beating as fast now as the snare drums that cease at the fall of the axe.

I ripped the ply off the frame, found the flimsy glass of the outside glazing and let rip through it with a kicking shoe, nearly physically sick with my heart beating like thunder; shouts from the nurses behind, crawling through the hole – hauling myself forward while they were hauling me back, across some jagged glass – and then I was out! I was climbing over the guttering, over the concrete rail to perch with my toes on a hold about five inches wide, and I let my hands go... then grabbed the concrete again! They were coming after me now, cautiously, from either side, a caution borne of the fact that my ass was swinging in the wind over a cement car-park seven stories up.

It was a drop of about 100 feet but I hate heights. It looked to me more like 150 feet. As I glanced down I saw a parking space marked "MB"... like the company "MB Games", or perhaps "Mark verses Boone" and I wondered – a flash sub – was that all it was about? A game? I had probably misread the letters "MD" but during that internal questioning some nurses pulled me over the guttering and then hauled me through an open window further up – onto a mattress where they injected me with a cosh. I struggled so hard a bed leg broke off. It was the first time I had been given Diazapam (Valium) that I knew about, and other very strong stuff besides. I faded to black for about three days.

Those times seemed to be a non-physical experience. I wandered about with no contact lenses in because I hadn't wanted to see my surroundings. I felt like a scrap of wood adhered to the surface of water, a piece of wood locked impossibly still while the water around it bobbed and rippled. I came to and found stitches in my lower abdomen that had been caused by the slash I had sustained while being hauled to and fro. Dad visited me. I had never seen him cry before. He told me he'd made arrangements for me to be admitted to Hays Grove Priory – again – if I wanted it, and I did. I had been in that black pit for about a week and I had to get out! Soon, I was empowered with new lenses and I heard someone announce on the radio that: "London Bridge will be opening at twelve o'clock," which I thought was referring to my retreat.

The decision to start smoking again was made, very quickly, because of the terrible withdrawal I had suffered in the I. C. U. in that place the year before. As the transport arrived I found half a cigarette lying about somewhere and picked it up. I got a light from a nurse as I was leaving and his lighter was surprising, like a small flame-thrower! I had the ready packed suitcase I'd taken to Wiltshire and there happened to be lovely clothes in it. Feeling laid back and thinking of the energy I was radiating as the ambulance headed south, the cyclic aspect of being in the same place in which I'd been incarcerated in 1990, did not escape me. As was my second bunk through those double fire-doors at the bottom of the I.C.U.

In WW2, it was considered a prisoners *duty* to attempt to escape. In late May, four days into that 'set', I decided I was going to make a break for it and this time I didn't need real fire to get out. The ingenuity of a psychotic can sometimes be an unpleasant surprise for a doctor and, once again, Murray was close. I was dressed and ready at half past six in the morning with my left lens in my right eye (for higher instinctive and longer visual range), took a deep breath, and then crossed the corridor. I smashed the front of the red "*Break glass in the event of fire,*" box, smacked it with the corner of a metal ashtray. The double doors snapped unlocked. The alarm bells were a sudden clanging; yet, as I headed outside, I still somehow heard a nurse shout: "Hey! Wait!" I didn't.

I ran up Prestons Road in the *opposite direction* to the way I had run in 1990. I felt freedom wash over me in the bright early morning sun. The plan was to deploy the address of the editor of Barker's *Nightbreed Chronicles* in Wembley Park, Middlesex, to maybe get him to take me in. I found a gate to some ramshackle farm buildings and scanned the area. All was quiet. No dogs. No movement of any kind. I opened the gate and advanced onto private land. There were barns around the place and bits of equipment, and farm machinery… the scent of diesel fuel and a musty smell of hay and dry rot. I walked into a wooden barn where I found an old truck. I tried the handle. It was unlocked.

I was happy to find a leather jacket, a thick rug, an old flat cap, and a pair of glasses with a negligible prescription that made a fine disguise. And also in the back I found boxes of passion fruit of which I took some. Then, I carried everything deep into the forest where I intended to hole-up for a few days until the 'heat' was off. I smoked a couple of Marlboros. Whatever happened, at least pride and matter-collectors wouldn't torture me as they had done the last time. I sat under the rug against a tree trunk. At about half past eight it started raining.

It didn't directly occur to me that I couldn't stay in the forest for long because of the weather. I had no knife to open the fruit and what I tried to eat had tasted lousy so I decided to make a move anyway, probably because of impatience as well as getting soaked. I headed down to the village and the shops were open and there were a few people bumbling about with umbrellas and raincoats. I kind of needed to piss but I ignored it. As I was passing a newsagent a man swooped onto the pavement on a yellow bicycle which he leant on the window. As he got off, and went into the shop,

I got on and rode it away! I had an adventurous feeling of achievement. I was wearing a perfect disguise and now I had transport!

I don't think it occurred to me to catch a train... not because of limited money but because the thought had most likely been *scu*-camouflaged. I suppose the idea may have flashed briefly through me. Maybe I had been cowardly – but in these circumstances actually getting on a train may have caused a severe fork in my destiny line. Further along, I popped into a tobacconist where I stole the last thing I really needed: while buying a pack of mentholyptus as a decoy I shoplifted an A – Z Street Map of London. Needing to piss quite badly I rode on through continuous rain and pulled up the bicycle into a parking lot. I tried the door handles of some cars and found an unlocked red VW Beetle. I was sopping wet and couldn't find any keys, but in spite of my time in Bristol I didn't know how to hot-wire it. Then the bike broke so I hid it in an alley.

I had to accept that my adventure was over soon after that, and in a most awkward and mundane way. Put succinctly, Barker's forces had 'bladder-locked' me. I couldn't release a drop and I felt bloated and miserable. In a phone box I called the nurses' desk at the hospital and then summoned a cab to get me back there. In the I.C.U., I bowed contritely before Doctor Mahendron and I was pleased to see him, my apologies born of relief. Within a week all the stainless steel ashtrays in the place had been replaced with those made of black plastic. We live and learn!

The processes of Boone becoming Bune had generated within me a belief with the strength of a castle, built with the unyielding stone of a thousand co-incidences. I had immersed myself so totally in the wonders and horrors of those existences that the possibility of becoming well seemed initially to be impossible. The psychosis had to be taken down stone by stone. So I got hold of some paper and thick marker pens and wrote colourful disclaimers that I tacked to the walls. I rejected the perception behind every twisted thought that had put me back in that I.C.U again, with some other happy expressions of encouragement. I wanted to get well. I read them regularly until I was moved out of that room. Then I didn't need to read them anymore because I had joined reality and come to believe in a simpler and happier existence.

My stitches were taken out, and in late July 1991 I was released from intensive care into a nice room on the outside. It was called the 'Lower Court Ward', much better appointed, obviously nothing like

a court at all – there weren't even any locks! I had two hic-ups before my rehabilitation could truly begin. One was a *sub-thought* three/way cusp: 'stay' (the sandwiches), 'go' (the Walkman), or death (the rope) and I survived a half-hearted tussle with the rope – typical of me! The second hic-up was an anxiety attack while I was on leave at a religious Fair. I got so flustered in the heat I'd had to dunk my head in a bucket of water that I borrowed from a "Throw the Sponge Stall!" Returning from the event I asked to go back into the I.C.U, feeling terrible and laid-up in a simple withdrawal room with a naked décor.

About a week later I was back to the beautiful bedroom with its plush furniture. There was a window with no restraining bar facing the garden, and a lovely plump duvet with a happy yellow cover. Entitled to go in the garden whenever I wanted I joined the others in the sun. I was happy, I was on a prescription of Lithium Carbonate, a blood build up 'salt' that I was told would get me better. I read a little, sunbathed a lot, and listened to my pocket stereo. Sometimes I'd notice a new song and walk down to the music shop in Hays village where I'd usually buy it on vinyl. There was a turntable on the stereo in the upstairs lounge. I played "Blue Lines" by *Massive Attack*, "Monsters and Angels" by *Voice of the Beehive*, "Winter in July" by *Bomb the Bass*, and others. It seemed I was becoming passionate. I wept listening to one or two of those records, good emotional healing as though I was a flower being lovingly watered. There was an atmosphere in that place; well being, a happy anticipation, things to do. I was a pot of rich earth, needed to cherish a flower of my own, and then I found a rose of dark red petals called Beverley. She had been through depression, and she was then almost well. We talked. She was twenty eight – six years older than me – had raced cars, and had a power position in London as an accountant at Reuters. Yet my desire to be her man was hidden. One afternoon after a shopping expedition in Bromley about six of us went into a café. We got coffee and then I suddenly I realised that Beverley and I were looking at each other – and we were smiling!

After that, sitting in her room talking to her about Barker, and art, and black miracles for hours, she told me of her pets. She had a rabbit called Bunny, a bird called Birdie and two tortoise-shell cats called Poppy and Lucy – and after the quagmire I'd been through this was good. Soon the stories were through. If you'll forgive me for saying so the stories didn't dry up, they got wet. We began to kiss, and cuddle, and I don't recall when this intimacy began but it was magical. As were the facts that she'd been seeing her last boyfriend for eight years and his name had been Richard also, and that she had a small house in Colchester! *Destiny Point* one might say!

She was tall and slim. She had long eye-lashes and brown eyes like mine and long straight dark hair. She was discharged from the hospital before me. I won leave to see her but that first weekend she had to cancel. I was upset but I saw her during the second. She picked me up in her car. We slept together... On some occasions we went to see a movie, or a drink in Greenland's Vodka Bar (I drank soft drinks to not risk going soft anywhere else!) or go dancing to 'Jungle' & 'Drum And Bass' music at *Too Too's* nightclub. We sent cards to each other, usually of rabbits or cats. I loved buying her cards. She wrote such lovely things to me. Since school, for my entire life before 1991, I had always signed off my letters with: "Lots of love," which became kind of limp and childish compared to what Beverley wrote. She wrote something I hadn't read before, that was simple and beautiful: "All My Love". I was discharged from the ward myself in August that year. I had become healthy in body and mind, and was deeply into reading a novel called "The Stand" by Stephen King, his extended version. I had a prescription of medication that I wanted to continue taking, my own creative writing to return to, and love. Yet after all that had happened, the most unlikely fact of all was that *I was alive!*

CHAPTER SIX: *1991 - 1997*

Sometimes I stayed at Beverley's where we ate vegetarian meals and swallowed our medication with white wine. I usually went outside to smoke. Her house was small but it was a nest that smelt of womanliness and soft carpets and warm cats. She returned to work, used to slip out leaving me in bed under sleep rapture until about 11am. Our sex was similarly manipulated. I lost my virginity with no fanfare of trumpets in about thirty seconds. I accepted *attack sub*-thoughts that it was disrespectful of me to watch her get undressed so I was always the first in bed with my lenses out. The 'base-controller' was terrible. She was the first woman to return my love in a mature relationship but maybe I didn't know how it was supposed to feel. Maybe I had never experienced that comforting warmth radiating through my chest. During the two and half months we were seeing each other I never once saw Beverley totally naked. What little I did see, when coupling in the darkness, I thought looked like Kate and I told her. Like smoking while she was out, it built resentment.

I used to sit about reading Stephen King. I didn't go out. One day Bev smelt smoke when she got back from work and said: "I see you've stunk the place out again..." and then she asked me if I had gone out. I said I hadn't. Although she didn't appear pleased I suspected that she had been acting a little. That perhaps she was packing a pistol with our relationship in her sights and was collecting my shortfalls for ammunition. Her bullets, like my poor sexual performance, were reasons I was mostly not aware about. "What, you never even went out *for a walk?!*" I knew we were sliding away from each other yet I felt impotent to halt the breakdown. It was as though I was watching a beloved building being demolished.

At the end I took the initiative one afternoon and rode round to Beverley's on my scooter for one final bluff. I had her house keys in my hand. I wanted to give them to her *before* she asked for them to try to undermine the control she had between us. But she simply took them and said: "I'll still be your friend..." Outwardly bitter I told her I didn't want a friend, I wanted a lover. Then I left the house with as much calm as I could muster while attempting to contain the destruction of my inner-self. The endless question "What if?" shouldn't apply. Barker and the enemy contributed to taking her away from me. I never saw her again.

The side-affects of Lithium sometimes jolted me awake at night hearing strange noises, with a taste like piss in my mouth and (when I turned the light on) everything I saw was green. I came off it voluntarily because I didn't think these weird and disturbing affects could have been caused by anything else. I was re-proscribed one of the older 'common neuroleptics', fortnightly injections of Modecate. I did group-therapy four days a week that made happy stories for my parents. When you begin to feel therapy is a waste of time you are probably ready to leave. To begin with the interaction was strengthening, like pushing bits of paper into the surface of oily paint and wondering how the pictures would come out. And through this skill – called 'marbling' –, which we actually did during an art and craft group, I imagined art was boosting me beyond the stigma of my diagnosis. I was leaving Barker and those 'long dark nights of the soul' behind. And a few of those pictures, though made in an automated kind of way, dried and were pretty.

I grew beyond the Day Hospital. My ego needed more than the groups had to offer. I felt the therapy experience had become kind of degrading so I rested my laurels back into creative writing to feel 'special'. Once I left the hospital I started negotiating with my father to rent a flat. He owned a lovely place in West Mersea High Street. My prescription of Modecate is actually a part of the dreaded Chlorpromazine family but I couldn't feel it doing anything, so I continued taking it so I could collect sickness benefit. By the late Spring of 1992 I moved into the spacious top floor flat, that was above a restaurant: fitted kitchen, two bedrooms, a huge sitting room with broad East and South facing windows – it was huge! The colours I selected were bright yellow and a kind of pink that isn't actually called 'pink' but something like 'salmon'. Anyway, I settled in and the place was destined to be the scene of some incredible parties.

A driving force within me, along with almost everyone else in the human race, was intoxication. During years the most rebel I had been was in a private school, so I rebelled later and wrote to counter any guilt between the first joint and the last bottle. My gay cousin Mike and a couple of hospital friends met regularly on Friday nights to drink several bottles of wine, the red Bulgarian stuff that carries you off to dribble land while eating your stomach lining. I found sniffing Amyl Nitrate and drug use enjoyable. My sister's 6th Form friends grew into friends of my own. The flat became Party Central.
I grew my hair long and wore denim jeans almost every day for the entire decade! I was strong as a rock and as crazy as doped yoghurt with a thread of slot machine gambling running through it all.

Between the winter of 1991 and the autumn of 1994 I was a 'raver' and went dancing regularly. The events had titles like "Mind Warp" and "Destiny" and some were over nine hours long. I first tried amphetamine "speed" on one of those nights, a few dabs of a friend's stash on a moistened finger tip. I liked the cushion of energy it leant me and within weeks I began to snort the powder through rolled up bank notes. Through *push-subs* and an amphetamine mind-warp I grew into what some might call a 'sexual deviant' – I occasionally wore women's frillies! You may think writing this is unnecessary but if a memoir isn't part confessional then it may fail. It was my way of merging with a woman: close to *being one* and being *with* one. During rare nights I blow dried my hair and used to 'podium dance' in the flat. Through drugs my female half was allowed to overtake the male to candle-lit music by such albums as Kate's *"The Sensual World"*, Deep Forest '1', and *"Mind Fruit"* by Opus Three. I'm not homosexual but it felt good to have my gay cousin as an audience for these intense experiences. We shared over two grams of speed, an 8th of hashish (sometimes smoked raw) with snorts of nitrate to put me into that place where I could reach, for brief moments, into the warm mystery of femininity. In a non-tactile way I became both Mike's missing boyfriend and *my own* missing girlfriend simultaneously! And I got away with this madness because I had my own space!

I would learn later that much of this behaviour was *scu* driving me to mischief. With no base-control-set and fully confident flirting, without my humour strangled and my ego strong, I might have taken dozens of lovers - in another life. During these years I was being driven through a kind of retro-active smear-campaign so that when it suited them one day I would become known as 'love gone wrong'. My reputation was being destroyed *years in advance* of becoming a Defender in the telepathy conflict. Once I sniffed a gram of speed up one nostril and another gram up the other in under a minute and was proud of it. But my brain often felt shitty because they twisted the affect – such as alcohol rapture. It's likely that I have known only once or twice how a few drinks are supposed to feel. I enjoyed this behaviour. I did. But how many choices of my own did I actually have?

My parties were arranged with excitement and sometimes verged riotous. I made solid friends at these events. There was little damage and trust allowed me less to worry about. My substance consumption felt like going down a ski-jump at night with sunglasses on ('speed' accelerating the speed) and rocketing off the end without ever really losing control. It is logical to assume that although what is intoxicating for one person may not be for another, almost everybody is addicted to *something*. I think this assumption is correct to differing extremes: one can't sleep without chocolate, another can't sleep without liquor. Some can't awaken properly without a cup of hot sweet tea and others are consumed by the mad desperation for a sniff of cocaine. I have what some people may call an 'addictive personality' and as the years passed the moral boundaries of what substances I would or would not take were pushed forward. Many a rebellious youth smokes cigarettes at twelve, white cider at fifteen, hashish at seventeen, LSD at nineteen, and who knows what other horrible shit can happen after that? Like those hideous LSD 'marples' preventing me from taking it after 1991 a user like me doesn't usually give up a drug unless their backs are against the wall.

At some point in 1994 I went to an outdoor 'rave' on cold mud in drizzly fog. I washed down half
an 'Ecstasy' tablet and started to feel sick. Shortly after that I took the other half and felt weak and weird and nauseous. I stumbled into a Porta-cabin toilet and puked up through the hole in the seat with the moon reflecting off the shit. I never did 'E' again. I have smoked a little heroin twice, which felt like I had a head full of ground glass. The last speed I took was in October 1996 because it didn't have the desired effect I had come used to expecting socially. The last hashish I ever smoked was on December 18th 1998 because it made my brain feel like it was full of fibre-glass and when had I purchased the stuff the night before I had thought my head was going to explode. But in the early part of the decade the flat on the High Street was a place that proved exciting for several years.

At the door, in the spring of '94, I suavely kissed the hand of a young woman coming into an event who introduced herself as Heather. She had a nice shape and long curly red hair. She sat with a friend. Although I caught her eye sometimes (we smiled) I didn't realise she was attracted to me. A gallon of red wine later, towards at the end of the night, and I found myself doing a puppet-show to an audience of seven people on a similar wavelength to me. They were stoned and drunk also. One had passed out! My show was animal magic and incorporated two slippers, a walrus and a rabbit. I burbled a lot of funny gibberish along the lines of "Walrus chats up Pink Bunny at the night-club and they go back to his place for a shag…" but it also turned out to be *animal magnetism*. When the others had gone off to sleep somewhere else, Heather stayed behind. She was lying in a sleeping bag by a night storage heater that didn't work, and it was cold. When I asked her if she wanted to join me in my bed she said "yes!" and it was as simple as that. The next day I needn't have worried that I wouldn't recognize her at our second meeting. With that volcanic eruption of hair she was as unmistakable as a red Post Office box! She loved to talk and we started dating. It was a life change.

After I wrote <u>The End</u> on my first novel *"Necronomicon"* I began a new investiture of my maddest dreams into fiction. Engineering my destiny into this new project that I called "*Armageddon*", it was intended to be a transposition of Barker's mythology into a 'realistic environment', utter catharsis. The writing was good, and fun to produce, but in its dependence on Barker's myth it would later prove unpublishable. Yet during its creation Heather was proud. She believed in me. I wanted her to read *Cabal* but she knew of my suffering and had no wish share that perspective. As far as I know she never did read it. Our sex was good, and however dubious the parties, it seemed like a full life. Yet my secret beliefs remained unquenched. I often felt within me the presence of more undiscovered. So I needed something else, or *someone else*, to confide in and put me on a new learning-curve.

I believed telepathy through music connects like electricity through water. When telepaths were on the radio they could hear (and maybe even *see*) my imaginings, but I could hear only the public broadcast. One night there was a new DJ on Radio One, and I was swept away by her name, a woman called *Charlie Jordan*. This name had special unfathomable connections that, with massive *push-subs* was like a laser piercing words in the darkness: "Come to me, you know me!" I listened to her show and found myself enjoying her voice. I connected and jumped in over my head; thoughts broadcast to her as though I had been with her forever... and some could have said that was true!

I wrote to her the next day. It was an exciting letter full of happy recognition and thus I found the fulfilment I needed: a material plane relationship with Heather and a mind-life relationship with Charlie Jordan. The third person, whose work I had been following closely was, of course, Barker.

To love someone and be jealous of them simultaneously is likely with a role model. Meeting the celebrity face to face and seeing them surrounded in the merchandise they have generated out of nothing, out of their sweat, is evidence of achievement the amateur is inevitably desperate to emulate. But how could the fan know that an Artist with a capital 'A' is born to greatness in the latency of telepathy? Given a pass to a mind-life on a silk lined escalator instead of a greasy ladder? For many the real ticket is not to be found gasping up that ladder but through telepathy and the overwhelming effectiveness of its scapegoat – mental illness! We are a war-like species but without this weird form of communication the world probably would have destroyed itself long ago. Just excuse me while I take some more medication!!

I wrote Barker some letters and he wrote back twice, the second time after I had jokily threatened to punch him on the nose if he didn't reply! Finally I met him in London around April 29th 1995. He was signing his books in a pub in Tottenham Court Road and that morning I dressed in a neat suit and rode the train into the city feeling pride and excitement and dread. I was carrying with me the only complete version of "Armageddon" in existence. I still don't know how that could have happened. Standing in the queue I spoke to people from the Royal College of Art, an interesting bunch of make-up FX students looking for work experience. It seemed to me that everybody there wanted something more from the man than just his signature, including me! I wanted his permission to publish my novel because it featured the consequences of a transplantation of "Cabal" into reality with Barker appearing as himself in a 'genuine' scenario. The two halves of the manuscript weighed heavily in my bag. At about five past one we saw him walk through the crowd like an exquisite Faberge egg passing by us on a conveyer belt. He went into the pub. Half an hour later I presented Parts One and Two of the

"Armageddon" novel bound neatly with cellophane sheets over the cover art. The first was a self-portrait I had taken in Hammersmith.

About it, he asked: "Who's this woman?"

"It's me!" I retorted. I wanted to stick it to him with a pencil or something, but in spite of dark fantasy or anger I don't think I'll do anything like that to anyone, ever.

"I remember," he said... "you're the guy who threatened to punch me on the nose aren't you?!"

"I'm sure loads of people threaten to do that," I answered. There seemed to be a kind of odourless smoke surrounding him that would later obscure my memory of his face.

"They don't, actually, I'm a very nice guy."

He asked me which publishing houses were considering the book and I watched him flicking through sections of the manuscript with a randomness I had seen before: absorbing sentences with 'K' linked synchronicity? In sum, he told me that his agent would send it to his office in L.A and then he gave me his business card that had his P.O box number printed on it. I went to the bar for brandy. That was over eight years ago. I never saw that manuscript again, and I never heard from Barker again either, for twenty-two months – until 1997 when he broke into my mind as a new voice of horror.

The writing of *"Armageddon"* wasn't only a matter of milking my secret life. Alike my relationship with Heather it was also an antidote to my addiction, gave me the personal respect that overcame the self embarrassment of playing fruit machines often down to the last coin. At least once I took Heather to an 'amusement arcade' (as many players called them, before the words 'Casino Slots' called in many more players) and I often lost more money in a session than Heather got in a week. She saw my addiction and didn't want to come in second to bits of machinery every time I was in Colchester so I gave it up. But like an alcoholic I didn't accept deep down that I would never play them again. I enjoyed sending time-delayed Faxes to Charlie Jordan's show and Heather had been accepted to university in Portsmouth and was going to live there in the autumn of

1996. I sent bunches of flowers and letters and sexy tapes to Charlie but I knew that if I didn't follow Heather down to Portsmouth we would most likely break up.

Between the two women was my fascination with Israel. I told Heather I may die there. Charlie's surname was a neighbouring country. Later I would come to believe that Jordan was a traditional enemy but at the time I had been ignorant of the friendship between the two countries created by the withdrawal of Israeli military forces from Jordan in 1995. Charlie's name rose from my sub-consciousness and manifested itself with an increasing interest in Middle Eastern programmes and news items. Compared to the stability of Britain, Israel is a strange place: terrorism... kibitzing in soap detergent factories... teenagers conscripted into the army... It all seemed very interesting to a young man who hadn't travelled far geographically that was busy in his own naïvety. And after I began to travel further, in my mind, I knew that if I actually went there and declared myself aloud to be a re-incarnation of Jesus, or the 7th Angel 'Bune', or a telepath 'Defender', I would most likely get committed into an Israeli mental hospital just as quickly as it took them to sign the forms!

Charlie's show *The Early Breakfast Noise* found me listening to the radio at weekends from four o'clock in the morning. Barker may have arranged the timing of it to tailor my sleeping pattern. I set my alarm sometimes, or stayed awake all night. Before the *scu* were instructed to spoil my loving interpretation of her voice I sometimes smiled to hear her. I lived for those tiny little hints that she knew I was there, knew I was listening. Such recognition would fuel the fires of war later. The misbalancing of my relationships put pressure on Heather. I had seen her wearing a brooch of a butterfly on her lapel as Lori had done in *Nightbreed* and trying to envelop her into understanding my 'secret life', I foolishly pressed the issues. I wanted her to love all of myself so I laid it out for her, even quoted The Book of Revelation; yet to believe that I was an angel was also to accept the destruction of hope and the end of life. It made her cry. I saw her tears of hopelessness and I realised that if I really did love her I would have to lie. So I tore up my presentation in a simple blast of psychiatry and told her that it had all been figments of mental illness, which it was. We went back to my parents. In the corner of my sister's studio was her collection of chipmunks that lived in a hutch as tall as the ceiling. Heather was still weeping but when she lifted up a baby chipmunk to look closer at it her tears became an expression of relief. I knew I had done right.

Before we moved down to Portsmouth I arranged for Heather to try teaching me Spanish. She did not know the true reason. It was because I believed that *Midian* was in Mexico. I wasn't adept at languages and sometimes her teaching seemed more like a kind of foreplay! I shared the flat with a young chef named Lee Harvey. I chattered on and on with my friends about Art and apocalypse, strange belief systems and the guidance of non existent 'co-incidence'. I wrote letters to celebrities, drew wild experimental *reaches* of gargantuan 'vicinities', and tacked the usual pictures on my bedroom wall. I communicated with Barker using the method of arbitrarily sampling words and sentences. I have actually done 'live' demonstrations of this ability before, perhaps a benefit of being *'between'*, being in the *Now*. If you fancy trying it out for yourself you can! Ask your question and open the text at random. Your immediate first understanding of a word is correct – even if it proves to be wrongly spelt when you look at it closer a second time. One of the most successful books I ever used for this was a paperback of crossword puzzles. Try to interpret the metaphors that are personal to you, but remember to be respectful: you may be talking to a Higher Power!

My secrets wanted to break out, an urge like the cracking of patterns and swirls in the skin of Boone's face when he changed into his bestial state. I tried to get a ten or twelve year loan because the world was going to end long before I had paid off even half of it! Lee and I and some of the lads went out on 'Nightbreed Missions' of midnight drunkenness and minor vandalism. I enjoyed the arcane taking me over. Lee seemed to become a believer, accepting facts such as that myself and a couple of friends had once adventured into Kent by car, found Kate Bush's house, and dropped three quarters of the *'Armageddon'* manuscript into her mail box! I moved out of the flat in the late summer of 1996 when Lee and one of his friends trashed the place. Before the turn of the century Lee had a picture of the monster *Peloquin* tattooed onto his back.

Heather got her 'digs' in a student house. She started her university course and I rented a basement flat that had views through the windows of brick walls. It was a dank and dim place with heating that condensed moisture down the walls, and Heather only slept there once or twice. I bought cards for the electricity meter that seemed to be reduced on automatic pilot. Heather made new friends and I started playing fruit machines again. We went to have dinner in the restaurant of a casino I had joined (just dinner) and shortly after that we split up. She had changed... I had just moved. I went into the casino often. I had been going out with Heather for over two years, and I may have 'let myself go', doing occasionally perverse things in the flat, and gambling, all to avoid facing up to my own relative loneliness. I played roulette with as much money as I could scrape up, and then I started cashing the £100 cheques. One night all I had to eat was a bowl of Smash potato. By October I was £1100 in debt at the bank. A post office clerk cut up my guarantee card and that cancelled any possibility of my winning back the position. It was over. I burned my casino membership and my father drove down and picked me up. Psychosis eased my financial disgrace.

By the onset of winter I was living back on the Island. As of old, I listened to BBC Radio One and sometimes sent them Faxes, sleeping in a small room painted yellow at my parents' house. When drifting off I sometimes heard voices calling my name. When your dream-self is connected to your memories, when you know you are asleep, it is called 'lucid dreaming'. In the knowledge that it isn't real and that therefore I could do whatever I wanted, I behaved like a flying sex pest, which would have generated a lot of discussion. To a telepath 'lucid' dreams can hold places to continue working, or to socialise, and for them it is another secret and serious reality. Between being awake and being asleep the calls of my name got louder. Within three days of the beginning of the New Year 1997 I became a full telepath, as I had hoped I would become half a decade before, but you should be careful what you wish for. With all horror and wonder that was to follow, I was now a full receiver of 'voices'.

CHAPTER SEVEN - JANUARY: 1997

The process started and finished in a dusty yellow bedroom that had a cracked plaster ceiling, a horror book and a Sony *PlayStation*. It had developed by prone states of rest when it evolved in transmission and volume. Getting off to sleep as a transceiver was initially difficult. Passing an invisible hand through my brain quietened things a little but I was advised not to and I can't remember why. It might have had something to do with dislodging equipment like *Reachers* but the dormant enemy, perhaps excited by talking about the worst aspects of my day, gave me a few minutes silence when I went to sleep. Apart from imagining music videos and feeding Ellie's chinchillas whilst listening to Radio One, I don't remember anything that happened that Christmas. By January 4th, I was using full 'eyes open' conversation and I had projections of other favourite Artists visiting me, including Charlie Jordan. I enjoyed meeting them. Before I went to bed I found other rooms in my parents' house for my exciting guests to sleep in also!

I stayed in the yellow room scribbling huge *Reaches*. As the days passed the visitors warmed me through the month with their friendly attention but I didn't know thousands of the other writers, painters, dancers, producers, actors, conductors, hardly any musicians and not many directors. In spite of passing 'O' Level English Literature a year early most interest I might have taken in literary fiction had been overcome by horror books. Faced with Shakespeare I couldn't understand a word!
I was named the 'Primary Artist' and although I had *The Art*, apparently, a force that Barker had written was the ultimate power, this responsibility didn't sound good. I couldn't know that I was going to have to fight from inside a narrow trench an enemy that had strategised and fine-tuned their arsenal of telepathic weapons for years.

Newly introduced guests were initiated into a group I called the *Harmonix* in a cosmic 'church' like a nightclub created using my imagination drive and two dance songs. I had recorded the music from Radio One's New Year's Essential Selection and made the environment using impressions of strobe flowers, UV light bars, and lasers, my new friends were enrolled before a Judeo Christian symbol of a Star of David on a cross. There was a huge Yin-Yang symbol revolving on the floor to be stood upon afterwards exchanging crackles of sparks from hand to hand. Some of my friends were probably acted by antagonists but it was a happy time, and important in regards as to how the silent majority perceived me. What lay ahead I would call my 'second life'.

The *PlayStation* was fun in spite of jibes about on screen violence. I sat at the kitchen table in the mornings to a dubious breakfast of a cigarette and a mug of tea discussing interesting items in the Daily Telegraph. The visitors accompanied me when walking our dog, Monty, or flew in a space ship into Colchester while Charlie rode with me 'on the back' of my Honda 125. Those cool bright afternoons in town I had believed I was walking hand in hand with my beloved Charlie! Barker advised me to buy a graphic novel by an author I had never heard of, Harlan Ellison. His book was called *"The Dream Corridor"*. I bought it. I was becoming accustomed to 'mind-life'.

It may have been said, being indoctrinated with false mythology, that I believed everything I heard with telepathy. In my own case I couldn't lie to the 'voices' because I sensed the proximity of embarrassment in my transparency. The enemy practised camouflaged attacks. Dream levels could be manipulated, such as the projection onto the First of black and white images called *intenseiform*. There were attempts to 're-wire' parts of my brain using single strings of tiny electrical spore, called *pneumas*, fired through the holes in my nose bone with a subtle *click*. *Pneuma* was a word perhaps chosen with educated sarcasm because in old English parlance *pneuma* means *spirit*. I thought the 'clicks' were a bodily verifier signifying *yes* or *no*. Barker and I fought the *cenobites*, the hideously body pierced demons revealed in the S&M horror of *Hellraiser*, which I thought were all too real. Barker taught me two secret words. In the construction of the Yin and Yang the 'S' shaped balancer is a revolving mirror called the *Deyaform*; and the containing circle he told me is called *The Asgaroth* – clearly spelt one letter at a time. I hoped he would teach me more, but this was not to be.

Around January 10th the crack in the ceiling of the yellow room opened and chunks of plaster fell to the floor in a shower of dust. Luckily I wasn't in bed at the time! When it was all tidied and vacuumed I began drawing '*reaches*' with a black fine-line pen. I was being listened to. I felt that I was useful. Kneeling at a table I sketched metaphors of how close we were – compared to the age of universe – now, to the end of cycles and new beginnings. I came to understand an aspect of *The Art*. It was Barker's honey trap because used too long use it was like the ring of power from Tolkien's *Lord of the Rings*. It killed love. I never asked for the thing but I was lumped with it and the longer I had it the harder it would be to reject. You could only be rid of it by crying. *The Art* suppressed such emotion by its very nature. I hadn't cried for a long time and even getting close caused a wracking pain in my forehead. Ellison made it clear that I was at odds with Barker, who expressed our inversions and reflections. We were enemies and we would have to fight for five things that we didn't have singularly, ourselves: a soul, a gender, Quiddity, an Asgaroth, and *The Art*.

Acting on hecklers 'shouting' *"Reach, Reach!"* I sketched an amazing re-working of perceived reality. If you can imagine this, another vicinity held something almost too gigantic to understand, called the *Incentimax*, a metaphorical cylinder stacked with 64 galactic plates including ours in a 'room' suspended above a lake of heavenly *Quiddity*. It rotated via a huge Deyaform, attached beneath and preventing the galaxies falling out (maybe a part of me) and kept within the cylinder by Asgaroth containment, (a part of Barker). We may have been in this position for a 'very long time'... The *Incentimax* is connected to a string of larger and even larger 'rooms' (such as The *Maxinity*, which I drew as having *more than one cylinder*) and then, at the world's end, the plates would fall into heaven like toppling dominos in a long-awaited *Niagra*. Barker would be left behind, stranded in a lifeless *Incentiform*... and because I would have disappeared to allow the galaxies free fall I had thoughts of doctoring this aspect of the *Reach* for a more palatable fate, since what could happen to me didn't look good!

Imagining *physical* options for the future was yet another mystery of 'pushed *Reaching*'. An old concept was that Charlie and I would share a motorcycle to the end of the world, go on the run and survive as long as possible... that the end of our planet was called a *Policy* (with a reference number I've long forgotten)... that if the telepaths delineating the forces of nature died simultaneously, in Hyde Park in 1999, a huge cosmic cog would rotate altering what those forces represented... that for souls who couldn't reject *The Art* there was the essence of a hospital for the treatment of failed Primary Artists, called the Ammorax, controlled by rasping nurses with long beaks... that in a different ending I would go to my spiritual mother's house in Kent with a code word to be allowed in... and inspired by history, I imagined myself being crucified with a nail gun; Israeli telepaths used to pop up occasionally from behind my bed to tell me to have it done in their cold season... news, or propaganda, to them? It was *all new* to me and I couldn't keep up with most of it. The nuclear destiny I had believed for so long would destroy us as a non-receiver may have changed. *I had changed.* Without any solid idea of how any of it would pan out I posted a sign (using forward projected imagination) onto which was written the expression *MYSTERY TRAJECTORY*.

If one of my guests created a problem I would use my imager to make them into an animal. I turned Sean Connery into a white Scotty dog and turned Kate Bush into a cat. I believed that Dr. Mammoud Mehendron was a telepath also and made him into a tortoise. Entertaining them all in the same house as my parents was beginning to feel like a crime. Mum and Dad knew nothing and when in close proximity to them I used to say in my mind, *"Chopping down to the Material Plane"* and then mentally change gear in order to talk to them. The mask I wore in the physical *Vicinity One* plane was slipping, wearing thin, as I was. More visitors joined me every other day and recalling all their names became too difficult. I feared exposure. The likelihood of my being committed to a mental hospital was looking increasingly likely.

However, much the bullshit steamed in those early *Reaches* they nevertheless retained a sense of being on the proximity of the *brink* of time, of stepping over the last final millisecond after eons into a new phase. I gathered that Harlan Ellison, who was an enemy to be and a friend of Barker's, was particularly bothered by this essence. I started reading Ellison's graphic novel "*The Dream Corridor*", but I couldn't understand a word of it. My concentration was in a cosmic blender so I abandoned it near the kitchen phone from where it disappeared...

Effective close-attention and memory are signs of alertness and well-being, and needed for strategy. I heard Ellison played chess with Stephen King but thought it was unlikely that even *they* had sufficient concentration to recall the lay of the board with only a shared *imager*. My own was hijacked often. I saw black and white 'hallucinations' of this other place I could hardly see, of telepaths sitting on a stack auditorium seats, flashing signs at me in the greyness of a place known to me then as the *Helter Incendo*. This was Barker's expression for the Earth. And there was a zone of subtle-bodies called *fundaments*, also, that I seldom saw – with any kind of 'eyes' – seated in an area Kate Bush had sung about on her last album – a vicinity called *The Circle of Fire*.

Sometimes I had sat with Barker at a table in the kitchen. We would 'talk' and he described us in those reflective terms: a cat and a dog, gay and straight, light and dark, and others suggesting a balance between us that simply didn't exist. He had been born seventeen years before me and was about as all-powerful as a living being on this planet can become, and he used this capability to supply people's thirst for reason and knowledge. He sprinkled everyone regularly with inventive myth. For years some believed that I altered the weather; in my happiness the sun might shine or in a depression it would rain from a dark sky. People wrote songs about it. He also said that in our case in the beginning we had been twins and that I was the elder, born a few seconds ahead of him. He probably said, as Ellison had hinted, that the continuing battle was a war between angels and demons fighting for heaven. And described between us another simple comparison: of *Good and Evil*. This last was the one that I needed to understand. The warning that should have woken me up to the horrors ahead – coming up fast – but unlike my nose ('verifyer') it just didn't click.

On and off on many occasions was the thought of rejecting cigarettes. As a receiver enemies encouraged me to give up smoking and to make an oath. Then they engineered unnatural withdrawal with machinations called 'matter-collectors', to make me start again. One collector was the equivalent, so I was told, of giving up a one-pack-per-day habit, and they could be programmed. Many had been known to drive me into the kitchen in the middle of the night for fruit juice or a can of coke. But it was smoking they reviled most. Long ago they may have themselves created the habit then left me to it, the extent of my addiction manipulated since. I'm no brain surgeon but it seemed that at times during the early / mid-nineties they increased the sensitivity of my pituitary gland so whilst smoking the carcinogens caused an increased surge of endorphins. I actually got 'high' on cola and normal cigarettes - that's what I used to take to gatherings while others got stoned on illicit stuff. Later on, this endorphin output would be decreased as a weapon. You think kicking the habit is hard? I've since told my family that if I announce I am giving up smoking this maybe a signal of approaching psychosis!

Good things sometimes happened to me, in the past, for doing good – not unlike feeling 'clean' and getting home safely after trashing those porno books in the South of France. I would progress. Eight and a half years later I got rid of some dirty videos and Charlie was pleased. I decided again to 'baptise' myself and filled a bath, immersed myself under the surface saying it was the River Jordan. It felt right, and the right time. Early in the third week of that month, while I was sitting against the sofa on the lounge carpet watching television, the enemy found their right time. Barker attacked me at around 7:30pm on February 18th. My part in the war had begun.

During the quiet while I was watching the programme a new voice started talking and it wasn't in my usual brain voice receptor. It wasn't spoken aloud and it wasn't coming out of the TV. It sounded like a demon. It was shocking, sudden and as scary as hell – spoke from a place deep within my brain claiming to be something called the 'Doctor'. Alike the psychiatrist character Decker – the true psychopath in Barker's novel *Cabal* – this claim utilized a truer and greater terror for me in those days. Far from the fearful funny stuff of Doctor Who, time was an adult's terror of an inescapable tunnel, a manifestation of consciousness stretching forwards and backwards through dark space forever. My hair was standing on end with terror. Soon the demon doctor said it was Satan, and when it finally admitted that it was Barker talking I could scarcely believe it. I felt so strongly towards him that I couldn't process this turnaround, so sudden and so venomous.

Knowing no other way to fight I used my *imager*. In one of my first attacks I visualized Hell. Marketing over the last few years has pushed the word 'MAX' to the forefront of shops and bars. Some prisons carry the colloquialism. I had thought that *Max* was another name for Hell. I pictured it as having increasingly terrible levels and used this structure as a deterrent when a particular *scu* had locked onto me demanding I go to Belfast: the *scu* of someone claiming to be a member of the 'Irish Telepathic Republican Council'. With no personal reason to go to the troubled North I showed the terrorist himself hanging in a room of blackness in a deep level of Max where terrorists might go.

I created the feeling of rainfall by imagining shaking maracas and I generated up to three *incentiform* cylinders at once to trap enemies in imagery that I thought was a capability of *The Art*. Whether it was my consumption of horror books or the manipulation of the enemy, I went into this fight punching below the belt. I pictured Barker eating his own dog and suggested someone burn him alive in an oil drum. Yet, believe it or not, I could not really hate him. Considering again the importance of opinion, these attacks probably weren't entirely my own. That burning idea was horrible and it was most likely based on our family's gardener carrying me away from a scare when I was little. As a boy of about six I put an empty oil drum on a garden bonfire – a sealed drum that had blown up with a terrific bang and a belch of black smoke. As I have already written I have memories of *pushed-sub-thought* in those days. Did they provoke this accident intent on a *child's attempted murder*? I write the word 'probably' when I'm not sure. Who knows the reason for that attack? *They probably* do!

I didn't realise for months that few of my thoughts were actually mine. Early that year I used to shoot into Colchester on my Honda, overtaking vehicles on blind bends and got away with my life. I called it "a sub-form of instinct". Once the war was underway there weren't many more fun trips into town to be had, just bad trips into my own mind. The enemy used to say "trust your instinct". I had none.

March 1st was Dad's 57th birthday. At half past six I rid myself of *The Art* by crying a single tear. I had taken so long to reject it could almost have been considered impossible. It utilized abilities I couldn't use, it was *Rapturer's* equipment and I had none. My mother came in asking me if I wanted to go to Dad's birthday meal, and I said soon. There was a colourful pain bunched in the muscles behind my forehead and I rolled about, moaning, and wept one single tear of frustration and was nearly sick. On the way to my sister's I thought that although this had been accepted, it may not have been genuine, may actually have been due to that stress of pain and nausea. Yet it was done. We went to Ellie's house where I joined the family at her table and adapted quickly to my knife and fork – soon after an imitator attacked me with a sickening opinion that I should be 'crucified, chopped up, and burnt'. Waves of horrified depression rippled through me and I felt this was sensed by the others. I could no longer see their smiling faces in the candlelight.

My mother's birthday is on March 24th. They guessed I'd be born in between and it happened: I was born on March 12th, the date of 'National No Smoking Day' at least twice while I was at school! Like other stable families our birthdays are smiley occasions yet I recall almost nothing of my own. I didn't go to Mum's because of a mind-life become rotten and uncontainable. In my efforts to evade hospitalisation I wasn't there to even *see* her. I remember receiving a fun *PlayStation* game as a present from my Dad and three days later I walked through the house saying goodbye. The enemy suggested that I commit the rooms and familiar furniture and ornaments in *High Acre*, where I had been raised, to memory but when I packed a rucksack for my escape I don't recall even putting in any family photographs. And anything I excluded from that bag I was not likely to see again. I couldn't bring myself to leave the space game; packed the *Necronomicon* manuscript, what I had left of *Armageddon,* maybe some bad poetry and a few clothes.

The *Hitch Hiker's Guide* theorises "people don't see what they don't expect to see" and I put this to the test when I hid my rucksack in the bushes by the front gate. I was to travel on the morrow. I was going to Ireland, after-all: to the South, to join my soul sister Enya. I doubt I slept long. Early the following day in all that cold brightness I dressed in black motorcycle leathers and went down to the kitchen at about seven. I was going to travel to a destination near Dublin and live with Enya in a house that I thought was called '*Green Acre*'. And never return. I 'went packing' as the Americans might say, carrying a decommissioned WW2 gun that I thought was a Webley '38. This relic was for bluffing – that's what I thought, belittling the border between actual danger and push-sub induced childishness. Enya represented *Water*. In face of this purity I had testing thoughts about kicking my important cigarette habit. Unable to, I decided to smoke perhaps one of the lowest tar and nicotine brands in the world, Silk Cut Ultra: 1 mg / 1mg, over 10X weaker than Marlboro red. My mother was in the kitchen getting an early mug of tea. I told her I was going out for a ride, recovered the rucksack, slung it over my shoulder, and drove away. Within the hour I was on the A12 in the rain to Chelmsford.

I arrived wet and dumped the Honda near the railway station. The helmet and keys were on the seat and I didn't expect to see it again. I got my ticket from there because it was less traceable than leaving from Colchester: there to Liverpool Street, the underground to Euston, Euston to Crewe, Crewe to Hollyhead – and finally a ferry to Donloughaire. I usually enjoy train journeys but this felt like I was having my head kicked in for over two hundred and fifty miles. The ticket cost me £65. I could have purchased a Return for an extra pound but I wanted to make it clear that I was committed to Enya – and to never coming back. But it would hurt.

So how could a force, as diaphanous as telepathy, be used to inflict physical pain? I have learnt that one method may be a kind of *voodoo*. Black rapturers, such as Barker, project an image forward of a physical object like holding a tennis ball in one hand and *meshing* the image of it with the other dimensional target – such as the brain within the victim's material body – and squeezing both to enhance pain and accuracy. I remember three possible examples and I'm not talking about dancing with headless chickens.

I had been asleep on my dad's boat when I felt a sudden stab in the heart. I jumped out of my bunk growling like an out of control affronted animal and thought it may have been a 'poppet' stuck with a needle. In early April '97 (Chapter Ten) a lot of the thick meat surrounding my inter-dimensional heart was ripped out – the love-growth I had built during my relationship with Heather – and I heard that Barker was simultaneously meshing and wrenching thick leaves off a cauliflower. That is exactly what it felt like. Towards the end of this very chapter I had an ache on the outside of my head caused by lots of telepaths meshing a ball in a 'brain squeeze' that made going to sleep difficult. On the night of the 16th February there had taken place more *voodoo* practised in a slightly different way, using methods partly *beyond* the physical plane. To talk his terrors deep Barker had allegedly used a piece of cotton tied to a pin pushed into an orange. He had spoken into the exposed tip of the cotton and his imagination did the rest. The enemy would probably say it was *rapture*, deny it was voodoo, but that's what these attacks sound like to me. There are other ways of causing pain but there is never any bruising of the physical body. Not on the outside.

The *Helter Incendo* is a grey place. S*cu* can go there but souls cannot. Most likely it is on the border with another vicinity called *The Circle of Fire* peopled by 'subtle bodies' called *fundaments*. *Scu* causes pain from the inside, and abused *fundaments* cause it from the outside – their pain transferred to my physical self, unintentionally, while they themselves felt nothing of the torture. Sometimes more than

<u>one</u> of my fundaments were assaulted simultaneously and I took it because I couldn't fight it. I felt like I'd been torn in half more than once. It was always going to be a *classic* weapon and I heard that *scu* could be raptured into fundaments – which were supposed to be vehicles for the soul to fly up to heaven – but Barker encouraged others to attack with them, his intention to raze the vicinity to the ground at the moment of apocalypse. Hence it was called the *Circle of Fire*.

The journey to Ireland was hard physically and hard mentally. I attacked Barker with images of melting him into a puddle I called a "buffoon stain". The no-smoking carriage on the way to Crewe matter-collectors drove me bizarre for a cigarette. My *fundament's* head was being pulled back and forth so it felt like my skull was being smacked on the table in front of me. There was a red and orange haze... glimpses of what could have been white bone, or an eye... and some talking that may have come from my own mouth. I was mostly oblivious to that also, as I was to anyone else talking, yet more *within* than *without*. I was ignorant as to how the other passengers may have judged me. None of them spoke. If I had been clear thinking I might have hoped their silence was due to my not being a bother to them rather than them being fearful of a man insane. The train drove on fast into the sunset, rattling never too loudly, juddering never too far off horizontal. It rolled on a kind of moving stasis that didn't seem to include me in my dislocated torture. But it *could* stop, independently of my mental alarm, or Pull the Chain In an Emergency, and soon it did. I disembarked from yet another train in Hollyhead and became a foot passenger on the fast ferry to Donloughaire. The journey across land was ending; the ending over the water was beginning.

After manoeuvring out of the terminal the engines turned over with a rumble that shook the entire vessel. Satiated with hot tea or coffee (another priority!), I explored the ship's shop and I was its only customer... or perhaps I just felt deliciously 'alone' amongst all those bright shelves. The bottles were quietly tinkling together as though mildly electrified and I bought two cartons of 200 Silk Cut Ultra. I wanted to be prepared and didn't know when the next opportunity to buy some would come up. I avoided gambling but after buying the cigarettes I didn't have much more than three pound-coins left to rub together anyway.

The ferry cut into the night with amazing speed. I found a balcony on the stern from which to watch the progress, caged in with metal bars. Britain receded leaving a wake for miles in a potential abandonment of freezing blackness. The propellers were kicking up a storm, two roaring washes that looked as though they were each a hundred feet high. The total effect of this thunder brought to my mind a *niagra* into Quiddity. At that pace it would be a short ride, and Enya would meet me off the boat. I believed that being with her might even *end* the war in its infancy.

As the ship moved up to its dock the lights on shore were illusory. They seemed to be moving to and fro through the cool windows as though *they* were moving and the ship was stationary. All stopped; a few gangways were plugged on like umbilicals. Carrying the pistol I passed through Irish 'customs' easily at about 10:40pm, perhaps worrying *less* about the gun than I should have done. Taking the strain for just a few more meters towards Enya's embrace I walked onto the pavement outside the exit, standing on Irish ground with the awareness that I was to make a home here – maybe for life.

With the telepathy 'accent-lock' I couldn't detect Enya's inflection when I was spoken to. For certain she wasn't there. I felt like I had been waiting for a movie to start for several days, and it began to dawn on me that the main feature film may never start; that the horrible journey might end in a worse nightmare to come. In the pools of lamplight in the car park I was like a balloon balanced on a fence of razors. Enya and her driver Roma spoke to me in my mind. They gave me a feeble description of their car and told me to find them at the far end of the tarmac. I couldn't find them there either.

All the vehicles were cold and empty, like my reception, so I moved out into the road. With the return of that ancient familiar randomness walking me I trudged down a ramp into another car park. It was small, a couple of dozen feet underground, and dry.

I may have considered sleeping there yet to admit that I would never see Enya because I had it in my mind and that this night was all there was. If she didn't bring me to bed, out of this cold tonight, she never would. Not defeated yet, I picked a scaffolding pole and made threatening gestures to a car windscreen. Either from myself or the Irish came up the idea of 'proving myself' by sticking this pole through the glass with a loud shattering *bang* that would have echoed back and forth, my heart racing. It was reminiscent of the night I was arrested in London, partly why I would never do the like of it in such doubt. But mostly I just felt like an idiot. I put the pole down.

After a time on the 'fence', teasing myself with ill-defined possibilities, I heard footsteps and a uniformed security guard walked down into the parking bay. I felt like the trespasser I was. He came up to me and asked a few questions. Back on the road I felt like a cardboard box that had been shoved out of a storm-cellar into a cyclonic depression. Another part of me was fed up with all the inactivity. I hadn't given up, and I needed to move, to do. Time was passing. With midnight coming I paused at a round-about by a ditch and withdrew the two cartons of 200 Silk Cut. I had it in my mind that smoking was the real issue preventing our liaison. So I told Enya I would give up, that I would throw both boxes of Ultra into the ditch if she just came and collected me. There was no physical response.

Walking into a built up area, maybe the outskirts of Dublin, a contact lens was dodged to the edge of my eye. The enemy had burnt my *fundament's* eyes during sleep for years, thus my own eyes. I used to wake up with them red and sore and dry, and to this day, inclusive of my usual waking routine, I immerse my whole face in cold water. Prepared for being a *Defender* before I was born, the design of my body may have included bad eyesight so that I would wear contact lenses because the majority of *scu* have only one eye. *Scu* see monocularly from either side. So with practise I could have looked clearly through one lens whilst emphasising the docile eye so no one could see at all. The other idea suggested in Chapter Two is that the fuzzy commonly non-dominant eye is chosen for the enhancement of equipment such as a battle grid – machinery like visual verifiers, energy levels, or adrenaline indicators – and other such James Cameron's stuff!

Standing in those urban shadows I had thought the lens had slipped for a reason. I had thoughts of sneaking about – unable to be tracked – but nothing happened. It was a dry eye, that's all. I used ambient light and spit in a car wing-mirror to push it back into line, then walked on. The situation was losing its potential: after midnight; quiet. A happy person can carry more weight for longer than an unhappy person and my back was aching like I had taken a bullet in the spine. So followed the ultimate verbal destruction, the worst possible statement in the circumstances: When Enya, or her imitator, said: "I'm going to sleep now," that was it. I was not in bed with her then and had to accept that I never would be. I was hundreds of miles from home with nothing to eat, virtually no money, no transport, no return ticket, and I didn't know a soul. There was only one place I might be able to find a bed without cash or a card and that was if I was lucky. I scored an address from a phone-box and called a hire cab to take me there. At about 1am I was dropped off outside the front doors, and on the early morning of March 17th I got tucked up and slept in a warm room in an Irish mental hospital. *Asylum* is a safe place.

I awoke with less trepidation than you might have expected. It had been several weeks since my last Modecate injection: sixty one months had gone since last a psychiatric tablet had passed my lips; and six years since I had last been admitted to such a ward – at a time when I had actually *wished* to take the treatment – but not in Ireland. Here my campaign of drug re-distribution would naturally take over and inspire brave acts. The indisputable proof of telepathy and my part in it as *Defender* had been verified with a wealth of jargon and tactile evidence. There was nothing wrong with me that needed to be recovered *from* so the treatment was re-distributed: out of windows, down toilets, into bins. I threw it into any vacuous hole where they were out of body and out of sight. I believed that enough of that stuff could drive you crazier than everyone suspected you were, that since gaining those endorphin 'highs' merely from common legal cigarettes I must have a very delicate brain. I was susceptible to the damage *that could have been* had I taken large doses of anti-psychotics since 1990, but that hadn't happened. In Hayse Grove in late May, 1990, a force from upon high had saved me from the horrors of overdose.

As in most mental health units with average security, by which I mean the main exits are locked but the staff call inmates "clients" and rarely restrain anybody in sound-proof cells, socialization is expected and rewarding. Meeting someone new there are none of the usual proprieties of the outside world; it is a sub-group so making friends is easy. Sharing your smiles or woes can aid recovery from whatever shit-storm put you there. I talked to fellow patients. I don't remember not enjoying the Irish accent, which has a haunting resonance to me, but most of my conversation was interior.

I had long suspected that Rik and Sal, our friends from Wiltshire, knew I was 'special' so I wasn't surprised to learn they were themselves telepaths. I had never intended to return to Mersea but I was going to be taken back in a hand-basket, soon, and staying away from my parents needed to be solved. Escaping hospitalisation and drug enforcement that 'home' represented was a driving force easily manipulated by the enemy. Rik offered me an answer to the insurmountable cliff-face of my parents' ignorance: killing them. Driven by seamless *scu* pushed-sub-thought, I said "yes" so Rik started driving to Essex. Soon my parents were revealed as also being telepathic. I believed it all!

The plot twisted and turned from my bed. Later on I directed Rik into the house where my Mum and Dad were hiding in the attic, terrified... then Rik couldn't do it, and he drove away. In my mind I saw a Cyclops, perhaps a figure of law, asking me questions about what I had hoped to gain from this crime, figments of an imagination out of control. I had only been fighting for a month and I remained new to it. I was upset with forces I could not identify and my parents were easy to condemn. I had been blaming them for a lot of my problems for years. But I couldn't have been insighted to murder if I was psychologically well. I never experience rage but the feeling of something being *right* and something being *wrong* can be all-consuming also – and <u>contrived</u> by multiple independent selves. In Ireland my thoughts had been so *pushed,* and it was the only time I have ever entertained the idea of murder. I doubt I ever will again.

I met a fellow patient who I believed was a chip off Enya's 'old block'. The enemy got me thinking that she was a poor mentally ill substitute for her *originator*, but she was a nice girl. The enemy was engineering a sense failure, of being on the wrong destiny line, but I never dwelt on it if I wanted to move forward. About six days later I had to say goodbye. I should have taken the girl as a pen-pall but I couldn't see any point in exchanging addresses because I didn't expect to see her again. My sister's boyfriend escorted me through Dublin and we got onto a plane. It was St. Patrick's Day. We flew back across the Irish Sea and as I looked back I left my brief friendships, and Enya, and the evaporating ghost of all that could have been, behind.

With hospitalisation on hold I visited a friend. It was always a cryptic pleasure to see him yet I hardly ever did. He was the closest man to an 'Air-Gate' I knew, named Tim Herring, and his forehead 'signature' was such an obvious block he hardly even needed to wrinkle up for it to be visible. We discussed my situation, him with the thinly veiled metaphors expected, and he actually told me that his tribe are the *"Hoovids"*. It is a name blatantly similar to that of the famous brand of vacuum cleaners. He gave me a book to read called *"Adventures of a Reluctant Messiah"* by Richard Bach. It was a thin novel with an easy style and I started reading it looking for a symbolic prophesy of my own life in the book – seven years later, and I was doing it again!

Chelmsford police contacted my Dad. My bike had been found and it was intact. I was pleased and we went to pick it up. Shortly afterwards, I ran away from *High Acre,* again, and went to a district called Eight Ash Green where Heather used to live. On March 27th I moved into the flat of my old friend Lee, and his girlfriend Jo, where one of the most horrendous experiences of the entire war took place. Shortly after that a new album by my favourites, *Depeche Mode,* was released. They called it *"Ultra".*

Telepathy was my preoccupation, my cause, and my life. It supplied meaning; yet the meaning that the enemy wanted me to have. I believed everything I heard. Good comments were rare, and I had sub-conscious questions such as why was I fighting alone, and why did it seem so many people hated me? These weren't articulated. I was on a learning curve in that youthful one bed flat over which the enemy had complete control. While Lee and Jo were out working I went into the fight in their living-room and it was a tight corner. I faced a sickening manifestation, different to Barker himself, yet another true master of horror: Terence Stamp... and the incessant unstoppable 'justice system' of the *Cusper*. In this example my re-distribution of drugs proved to be disastrous. If I had accepted sleeping tablets in Dublin this approaching nightmare wouldn't have even come *close* to happening. I accused the enemy of attempted murder, later on. That may have been naive.

The sleep deprivation started around the night of 29th March. I rolled around in my sleeping bag, fumbling in the semi-darkness, and I couldn't get to REM. It was mildly disturbing. Day followed night and no morning was new. Each was a gradual disintegration into worsening anxiety. Torturer of Los Angeles, Terence Stamp, was an evil of old whose deeds had apparently been so terrible at the end of the last 'policy' he had lost himself to them. He hadn't been able to eat and hold down all of his food in this life. And unfortunately for many he was equally sick in other ways. Barker had taken him into his sect against me, guided Stamp with myths and manipulations that were most likely bullshit. For my own part I wore jewellery signifying my side in this war, a silver cross and a Star of David hanging from a silver chain. Stamp lied continuously. I learned that he wanted the manuscript of my first novel *Necronomicon* because he believed in the proximity of sub-conscious *reaches* that he could use to avoid the same fate. I believed it was why I had written it in the first place.

I couldn't post him the entire book because nothing else could hold him back, so I took a pen to the task of making a deal. I wanted him to disengage his weapon, *'intenseiform'*, the projection of mostly disgusting B&W images, which I heard he had used on children. Bargaining, with the like of Satan, I made exhausting deals using *Necronomicon* to make time for what I realised I needed the most – sleep – which was also affected by something else, a pain in the head, the 'voodoo brain-squeeze' I wrote about in the last chapter.

I arranged for Stamp to hear one page of *Necronomicon* at a time, each night. An attack would result in my tearing it up. At the time, I thought there was a possibility it was the only copy anywhere and he called my bluff often. So instead of reading them I destroyed them. Over fifty pages later Stamp may have been less interested in the manuscript because of my flagrant disregard for the worth of my own writing. Days blurred into nights. Neither state was truly wakeful. I became too exhausted to continue the times set for bargaining and Stamp had probably been lying when he called my bluff anyway. Barker rounded me up in the flat, shouting: "Hate me! Hate me!" but I couldn't. I saw moving *intenseiform* one afternoon while I was awake, an image of a baby getting run over by the wheel of a van and I screamed. The nightmare was stepped up by April Fool's Day. My friends were home during the evenings but I couldn't bring myself to tell them what was going on. I was thinking about knives. My motorcycle was outside and I rode it to Vagabonds once where my conversation was stunted by a 'gut twist' but I never went to my parents, or to hospital, or to anyplace else I could have got help. There was a telephone in the living-room but I didn't pick it up until it was too late.

I used to climb out of my sleeping bag in the mornings saying I'd "just had a rest". In those days I attacked by visualising sticking needles into the underside of an enemy's brain, or with fire, or freezing liquid gas. I was so tired I felt like there was sand gushing against me from a pressurised fire-hose. My mum used to describe this exhaustion as being "too tired to sleep" because of natural serotonin, which incidentally can also be produced by certain illegal stimulants. At the non-existent mercy of a force called the *Cusper*, I was dizzied by a storm of 'justice' called *Helter Insinto*: the acceptance of guilt via the worse fate – of two choices – to lessen a 'sentence'. Lee and Jo were out while it mangled me.

Cusping was dreadful. The questions were accompanied by daylight hallucinations unfolding before my eyes making such horrible futures seem very possible. I sensed I had made the same mistakes before. "Beetle or cig?!" asked the enemy. "Cig!" I replied, so I was allowed to smoke. "Cig or shit?!" / "Cig!" / "Then shit! – Shit or a half soul in nullility!?" / "the soul!" / "Nullility or 'incentimash'?" or "worm" or "nicotine molecule" and so on, and on... for hours. Sometimes I hallucinated my soul as a small white thing in space. Often, after more botched answers, that didn't exist either, lost in darkness. I believed that the Air-Gate (which may have also been the *cusper)* couldn't deal with smoke or music so I sat on the sofa and had cigarettes listening to my pocket stereo... but it was too easy, of course. It didn't stop them.

There never seemed to be any good choices. I was having thoughts about attacking myself with a knife, the brave thing to do. I went to bed barely sane, restless in the hot claustrophobia of my sleeping bag. The room always brightened slowly. By 2nd April I was totally insane, got out of my bag and wandered about aimlessly with a contact lens missing. I told the attending telepaths in the bathroom mirror "I'll never need to sleep again;" and when my friends had gone out so there began the last delirium. What grip I actually had on reality had the essence of skiing on roller-blades behind a moving train – wanting it to stop but not by falling over.

After a mess of further cusps, accusations, and insults, the bright morning was eclipsed by a psychotic act. Suddenly I was in the kitchen, picking up the biggest knife I could see, and my wrist was like a tree branch as I began to chop off my left hand. There was more blood on the kitchen floor than I care to remember and after I hallucinated a white fish bone falling into it I stopped. Many tendons were severed but it could have been much worse. Nevertheless I needed oxygen while going to the hospital. It took over half an hour to get an ambulance to collect me. I had had to telephone them twice. I didn't see the injury again after transportation for any significant time until the bandages were unwound. In Colchester General the enemy piled it on without mercy, most likely consolidating their advantage.

The A&E department didn't look busy so I couldn't understand why it was taking them so long to see me. With the hem of my sweatshirt pulled down over the wound I got off the trolley where I had been waiting, and went into the hospital shop and stole a chicken tikka sandwich. I ate it and got back on the gurney. The wrist felt sticky, the ache dull. It was not overly painful but it was like a parcel with a bomb in it that had to be faced up to, and opened, later. After about four hours I was finally seen... then carried upstairs and prepped for surgery. Barker had said that a telepath cannot survive being anesthetised. A nurse took my jewellery. "Do you have a crown or a cap?" someone asked. Which I thought meant to a patient with suicide damage that they could supply euthanasia if it was wanted. I said a cap. I was awake with a little fear, yet also exhausted. The operation drew near and I said if I died I wanted to have a bed, and air, and my soft pillow 'Fred', a comforter of old that had the dog Fred Basset awake on one side and asleep on the other. I slid away... on wheels, wheeling... everything went black.

I came to 'a few seconds' later. I was in a bed with curtains around it. I needed a cigarette badly but there was a drip in my arm. It was linked to a bag of clear antibiotics hanging from a frame at my bedside like a sanitised bat. A machine on the nurse's station *beeped* every few seconds, which the monsters called a *cusper* because its noise was rhythmic and ceaseless. I may have felt fearful of a *'locked moment'*. I was intensely aware of sensate involvement with my own body: needing to piss, or itch, or smoke. The nicotine 'matter-collectors' were coming on strong but nowhere in society is less likely to entertain smokers than a hospital. I tried to go to the toilet but the enemy had initiated bladder-locks. I managed to smoke on a balcony, or maybe it had been on the ground floor, so I felt better for a while. My water-works were horribly stuck so I had a catheter inserted but even with that I still couldn't go. There may have been a discussion on the conventions of fairness verses sadism, which I didn't 'hear', but it would explain why the bladder-lock was resolved and released. I must have been taking night sedation because I did sleep.

The enemy called this place *The Ammorax*, like the surgical ward for treating the souls of people who couldn't reject the power of *The Art*. This was a place I never believed in 100%. Likely, it had been a push-sub at its conception, a false reach like a lot of other stuff I had drawn up in the yellow room in January. Days passed, dipping from sleep to wakefulness, to sleep, and back and forth. I can't tell you how the food arrived. I don't remember eating. I thought the clearly mental problem indicated by my wound was causing less sympathetic care, that since it had been self-induced it was wasting resources. Restrained by drips and needing to smoke, ever more desperately, and get out of that uncomfortable bed, about six days after my admission I pulled the needle out of my arm and ran down the ward with a cigarette in one hand and a lighter in the other.

I remember being rolled down to The Lakes feeling like a king, in a wheel chair. On arrival, I had the most delicious cup of tea and a cigarette for an age. Such relief is part of being in a mental hospital 'set'. I had tried to avoid being Sectioned but the *psychiatrists had me* and that first night I was given a yellow tablet of the 'common neuroleptic' *Meloryl*. I palmed it back to my room where I cracked open a can of Coke and swallowed it certain that the combination would cause an erosion of my delicate brain I called a *"tip"*. Nothing happened, of course. I went to sleep. At other medication times, I was routinely selective: dumped the *Meloryl*, took the antibiotics and half the *Zimmervane* 'sleepers' prescribed, secreting the rest in a pill bottle to prevent a repetition of the horrors that had put me there. Would my enemy attempt sleep deprivation again? If they tried to, I now had the pills to stop them. Another question was that since I had received antibiotic *tablets* as soon as I arrived at The Lakes, why had I continuously been on a drip for so long up at the General? I settled into ward life.

My room was clean and it had an optimistic atmosphere. My bed reflected a latent sleepiness even in the bright light of the day. For want of a home it became *my room* and I felt delicate getting under the bed covers at night when all was quiet. I was aware of deep breathing from every room. I heard it with my heart rather than with my ears, a knowing that all of us were sharing sleep. The nights were mostly dreamless. Days were for telepathy.

Terence Stamp was occasionally called 'Frank', as was the character who had escaped a doomed eternity in Barker's movie *Hellraiser*. Once or twice I was *intonsiformed* into Stamp's mind. If I imagined myself sitting in a room watching myself from the ceiling, or in a top corner, if I then disappeared from the image – leaving an empty room – then my soul would have been taken to a terrible place called the *Ziggurat of Ur*. This had been a temple of blocks stacked up in decreasing sizes, a sight perhaps of human sacrifice, in the city of Ur where writing had begun, originated in the wedges and slashes of *cuneiform* engraving. The ziggurat was represented by – and somehow *within* Terence Stamp's mind. Yet it was just a conceptual attack. I saw no bloody horrors and that was why *intonsiforming* was abandoned. I had other problems, anyway, issues developing the Defender I would become.

When I first got into bed to try for sleep I usually faced the vicinity that Barker had written *was the Earth*. It was a continuous presence 'somewhere else' called the *Helter Incendo*. I saw it with my eyes open: a black and white place, full of secrets and moot questions. I posted a photograph of Sharlene Spiterie (vocalist of the band *Texas*) on the edge of my bedside table thinking she looked like Charlie Jordan. Within three nights Barker's voodoo attack was taking chunks out of my left hand heart – in the folds of which he found maps of star systems and galaxies. In the *Incendo* Barker sat behind a desk and Ellison had a rack of deer-stalker hats that he used to eat one at a time if I did anything astonishing. Charlie had a *chaise-longue* near me and I had two Uzi assault pistols (the Israeli manufactured fire-arm) and kept them, like a bizarre Jimmy Saville, in the side of my armchair. With an idea poached from Sean Connery I ran down Barker's table in a military tank, but I couldn't defend myself when getting to sleep. In which event a force used to come to my aid that I never saw clearly. "Who will be your *quice*?" the enemy had asked. I don't recall supplying a name. I wasn't even sure what a 'quice' was, but whoever must have done well, for I did sleep.

The injury was ever present. Some afternoons I went up the road for physio. The therapist was a pretty woman named Mary Knot and her strong hands working E40 cream into my scar tissue felt lovely. She moulded surgical appliances for strengthening the repaired tendons out of blue plastic. One of them held each finger up straight yet flexible on individual elastic bands like some kind of a miniature guitar. I made jokes along those lines. Barker called it a soap-dish, possibly a general term that included another, smaller 'soap-dish' for night support. I began squeezing plastic balls and rolling sausages of different densities of coloured putty, but not for long. I never completed physiotherapy – didn't even get close – for two remarkably normal reasons. Two ingredients that can drive a man's life: for money and a good woman.

A client's 'income-support' used to drop after six weeks on a ward. Nowadays it is paid for up to fifty-two weeks. All the money you used to get then was sixteen pounds per week and it was a common motive for people to get discharged early. The other? She was called Sandy Delafield, a deliciously tall blonde of about thirty-two, undoubtedly a 'chip' off the late Lady Diana's old block. She was well spoken, pretty, and her blue eyes teased yet they were kind. I wore Mary's appliances less and less. Early spring was out there to be experienced – and so was Sandy!

Across the road from The Lakes lies High Woods country-park. There is a lovely forest with a lake frequented by the occasional duck or coot. Under that canopy of virgin green, Sandy and I walked hand in hand through the trees. In spite of our past we were both mentally quite healthy, like fish pulled out of an oil slick, washed, then placed into a tank of clean water. We kissed each other... and that may have been 'it' – except that the enemy wouldn't sit still for it. Once they filled me with sickness all throughout my innards as we hugged. I felt nauseous at the exact moment we were kissing in Sandy's room but I kept my stomach under control. The enemy did lots of shitty terrible things, but Sandy made me feel appreciated and happy. I looked forward to consummating our relationship sexually, soon, in her little house. I had a girlfriend now who was rescuing us both from the worst of our pasts to share a brighter future together. Barker's horror adapted quickly to these new circumstances yet the attacks done to me beneath his banner were tame compared to how they had been.

The surgical staff never returned my earring, yet I retained my Star of David and the silver cross, which hung heavy with meaning from my neck. In spite of causing trouble beside my armchair in the *Helter Incendo* I wrote to my beloved Charlie often and it would be many months before I would learn that then she was being imitated also. Sometimes, when my brain felt as though it had been soaked in corrosive acid, I hallucinated a small and transparent thing like a flea circus. It featured a moving roller-coaster and a big wheel that turned that I called "Mr. Stamp's Funfair". In the limited world of the hospital set I made new friends. One gentleman there, named Donald, bumbled happily around the wards laughing and talking, and Charlie liked him too. Hanging from a chain he also wore a Star of David and a Celtic cross: the truth; as is everything else I have written in this book. I sneaked into Donald's room and found a book called *Telepathic Sex* or maybe it was *How to Have Sex with Telepathy,* or something. Donald wasn't a genuine telepath but he was certainly a living indicator and verifier of my own beliefs. And on top of the pedal bin outside Gosfield ward smoking lounge I found a book called *Israeli Paratroopers*.

The enemy have said that I fall in love with any woman I kiss. Maybe in a few rare cases this has been true, to varying degrees, particularly with the undeniable existence of *push-subs*. I didn't want to care except that the enemy emphasised the worst points of Sandy. Although her teeth were a little askew and her breath had been known to irritate me I liked being with her when the enemy let me; I liked kissing her and I liked her to hold my left hand and stroke the lacing of tactile scars that so needed love. If cement had a life, my metaphor would be that my wrist was like a damaged pavement freshly mended and ready to be used, desperate for the reassuring feeling of people walking on it. Sandy was kind and patient, a single mother of an eleven year-old boy called Danny who was staying at her sister's in Cornwall. I visited her at the weekends. We had good sex. She was anorexic but paradoxically had a nice womanly shape and it was the first intimacy I had enjoyed for ages. The problem, basically, was that Sandy's 'ex' had stalked and tortured the minds of her and her son so badly that they'd had to spend many weeks barricaded closely together in the house.

I wanted to get out of The Lakes. The expression commonly used in those months was 'bunking it'. It is better to be poor and well, than rich and unwell, in most cases – but I left anyway after five and a half weeks with my benefit monies secured. I was still a long way from acknowledging that I was mentally ill because of so many years of undeniable proof, so I made pretence of glowing health to my Irish consultant. I bullshitted him until 18th May when he discharged me against medical advice. I went back to *High Acre* with a small supply of *Zimmervane* and a blue cotton duvet cover that I had taken from my room. It was lovely and soft. My parents understood my need for space now so Dad cashed up my trust fund and we went looking for a flat in and around Colchester, looking for a place to call my own that was far from Mersea.

Sandy and I drove South West to her sister's to collect Danny. "She's *sand*", the enemy had said, "*She's sand.*" It was a long way to Cornwall. On that first night we slept in the car. Moving on, the enemy moved on with me, adapting, lying, horrifying. My belief in their nonsense was leading me up the garden path into Hell. They said Sandy's relatives were a 'Deyaform family', a close-knit unit that ate together, got regular exercise, didn't smoke and liked sports. That I was invading their privacy and that I could never be truly welcome among them. Sandy's brother-in-law was a schizophrenic professional artist who painted pictures that looked kind of musical. Danny hated me on sight and his Uncle insinuated that Sandy and her son may have had an 'unnatural relationship'.

Sandy and I shared a cuddly bed in an attic room at her sister's where I decided orgasm might make *Zimmervane* obsolete! Near the following day I broke the underside edge tendon of my injured hand when I slipped my thumb carelessly into a pocket of my jeans. Even today the thumb remains unliftable. Most likely I'll get it put back together, but surgery in the General, *again?* As a receiver of 'voices', *again?* Fuck off!! Once or twice in Cornwall I had a beautiful vision of a rainbow over mountains with doves taking to their wings in the misty air. I thought it had been Barker broadcasting a pretty signal to me that I could or would die safely soon. Walking along the edge of a beach one afternoon we came across a grassy hillock speckled with rocks at the top of a cliff. Within moments the enemy were calling it 'calvary'. They said that in a 'policy' long ago the singer Cliff Richard had been me and had been rewarded for jumping off a cliff like this one to his death. Maybe they meant this very same cliff! I imagined a running dive ending in a bloody splat on the rocks below and walked on by. If future 'trajectories' could be represented in film plots the enemy suggested this one was to be *The Shining*. I did not accept that. I knew it wasn't likely we were going to be annexed anywhere in a raging blizzard anyway, not in England. Was Danny a re-incarnation of Hitler?

The weather in Cornwall was bad out there though, raining and cold on the third night when Sandy and I were relegated to the garden. I fumbled with my girlfriend in the darkness of an old leaking tent, *push-subbed* that we had to conceive the last soul out of the 'Guff' – or have the first baby of the Armageddon with no soul – those kinds of horrors. Rain poured through the holes in the canvas and I stopped the embarrassment with Sandy and apologised to her quietly. I didn't sleep much. No longer than five hours. We climbed out of the tent cold and soaked, and the message was clear: Sandy's sister wanted us out. So that afternoon the three of us got in the car and drove north east on the journey back to Essex. Feeling exhausted and obsessing about rest again I could see the shapes of people lying down sleeping in the sky. Both mother and son were asthmatic. I believed that car exhaust fumes could help them breathe easier...

Back in Colchester my Dad and I went to look at a clue to the place we would eventually buy. It was on the

Fingeringhoe Road on the outskirts of town in a place called 'Thornfield Court'. The rooms were laid out well but it was on the ground floor and it was messy, smelt of babies, and had cat scratches on the skirting boards. Yet we got lucky, finding another flat on the market in the same location, the size and lay-out of rooms very similar, but this one spotless. It was for sale by a lady schoolteacher. It had a good feeling in it and we could afford it. There was a lovely first (top) floor view from a red tiled building set back from the road along a winding path through a garden of rose bushes, with a honey-suckle tree soon to grow yellow blossoms.

The two main rooms had floor-to-ceiling windows that were each over seven feet tall and there was a gas-fired heater in the sitting room. Night storage heaters waited for winter tucked away elsewhere. The kitchen was basically equipped but would shine in the mornings in east-facing sunlight. The bedroom had fitted wardrobes and all except the bathroom had good grey carpeting and long blue floral print curtains that we had secured as part of the price. There was no 'chain'. We bought it at the asking price, a hole-in-one, and bought a nearly-new shiny Honda CG125 with the change, a blue trim and chipper little town bike. There was a sign on its fuel tank lending me a sense of eco-friendliness, saying _unleaded petrol only_. If it was running badly I would call it 'Ermintrude' and when it was running well I called it 'Ermine-scoot'! These were good days, yet Sandy and I loved on borrowed time.

When I stayed at her house I smoked as few cigarettes as I could indoors. My mind was in a twist about her asthma so I made arrangements with the enemy about how many I could actually have. Yet Sandy hadn't seemed to mind. If she _had_ blatantly said "no" I wouldn't have smoked in the house and often I went outside anyway. Characteristic of my enemy was the initiative to induce an oath that they made certain I could never actually keep. Occasionally they would instil an explosive fear of smoking that made even the act of lighting one seem brave, and instil guilt feelings hearing anyone else cough. Smoking drove the power of *The Art,* they said, and regularly employed lung/rapture attacks after which I would wake up coughing and go to sleep at the end of the day with lungs as healthy and fluffy as puppies, or twelve hours the other way. Perhaps more 'cat people' than 'dog people' smoke and Sandy herself had a jealous dog she called 'Lucky' that was a canine lunatic. Three in a bed only works for the sexually advanced and too far for anyone, when a crazed Jack Russel terrier gets involved. When Sandy and I were about to get sexy in her sitting room, Lucky would scrape frantically and sometimes escape like Houdini and come charging downstairs leaping and barking, jumping all over us with its fur standing on end! 'Lucky' wasn't lucky for anyone.

But Danny was the true third in the house and it was his breed of jealousy that killed our relationship.
Sandy told me that her son had once stuck a piece of cutlery into her. She had been smiling enigmatically at this reminiscence, her expression typically challenging. After her experiences with the boy, Sandy's sister had recommended he should be put into care. I suppose I wanted that also but Sandy wouldn't have considered it even if I had said it more than twice. I had seen them eat the same pitiful meals; toast, bananas. Sandy's illness had manifested itself in anorexia and her son's in angry tantrums. Traumatic experiences can be so emotive, so *bonding*, and I figured they both wanted to regress to that old familiar routine against Sandy's 'ex'. At the bottom of every mental illness are relationships but my opinion was moot.

When Sandy visited me I tried to feed her. It was a suggestion of the enemy that was met with hostility, which failed nearly every time. But she seemed to like my home. Since watching TV mostly against a seat on the floor at my parents I wanted to furnish the place as a 'floor flat'. There were patterned throws and bean-bags in the sitting room, and I enjoyed the most visually delicious sex for years seeing Sandy's nakedness in the honest light of day, our intimacy softened on an air-mattress on the bedroom floor. At night I used the stolen pale blue N.H.S duvet cover as a 'summer-time sleeping bag'. I had a gilded lamp on a low table, in there, casting shadows through a piece of basket weaving scrounged from a charity shop. There was a rug like Barker's *Weaveworld* in the sitting room, low tables and a corner shelf. The TV was stored in a cupboard. I had trouble patching together my stereo but when I managed it the sound quality was good. I loved this place. Even when the war became so terrible that it truly befitted the name *"Thornfield Court"*, after battles at my parents' house and in hospitals, I repeatedly went back. I was a slave to schizophrenia yet a master of my own space so I went back again and again into that pain for another *twenty two* more *months*.

CHAPTER TWELVE – <u>JUNE: 1997</u>

As a couple we sometimes shared excursions out of town. We visited a nature reserve in Fingringhoe during a warm day under a blue sky. The enemy asked what my idea of heaven was and I wasn't sure. Sandy and I also bunked it to a "petting-zoo". I love small animals and the place had a menagerie of them in a large enclosure with domesticated birds. It was funny seeing them strutting about with their beaks pecking the air with that alien kind of determination and aimlessness, and the cacophony of squawking and clucking got me into a pitch of high humour so hilarious I couldn't stop laughing till tears rolled down my cheeks! There was a goat also, with demonic eyes and a black pig snuffling about: unfortunately the enemy overlaid it with the word 'Zion', which freaked me out.

The song of the day was: *"You're not alone"* by the new vocalist Olive. It had a powerful emotive rhythm, a melody of epic quality, and I took the lyrics at face value, found encouragement there. But I was told that in telepath vernacular the word 'not' also means 'nullify' – ceasing to exist by yourself – "you're <u>not</u>, *alone...*" Hearing another tune on the radio called *"Love is the Law"* it was suggested that I should make laws but it didn't feel right. I didn't know where to even start! I learnt telepaths have a visual panel called *Data-Form* that was filling with laws from Lord 'K', Asgaroth of the Earth. The laws, developed every day, were a code of conduct based on doing whatever made me happy on a regular basis, yet I could hardly read them. It was like trying to hold up a traditional photographic negative and becoming confused with the light and shape of the scene behind it. I still accepted a coming apocalypse and one of the early laws stated that I should weep for the fate of the Earth each day: I didn't wonder then, what was my purpose? No clues. I hardly even considered the question. *Defender* is an expression I have developed in retrospect. Since coming such a long way to being healed I have applied it to myself, and I am writing this memoir as a war story.

Sandy was the last really good sex I shared. There has been no one since as fulfilling as her. When loving the sight of her on the air mattress I knew that others were seeing her nakedness through my eyes. The telepaths had been calling it "lessons in love" and I wasn't angry but in an honesty that typically damaged my relationships I told her they were watching. I didn't want anything to change. I hadn't expected much more than to make myself feel better, yet at the expense of Sandy's impression of my mental health. I used to ride my motorbike to her house, outside of town on the road winding through Friday Woods, and I would often stop off at an unmanned stall in the trees to steal a pot plant. Sometimes I left the plant on her doorstep for her to collect later.

It seemed that paranoia was compacting mother and son into their old, terrible yet comfortable, status quo. Sandy was back under Danny's thumb. Both were relapsing to days that neither could let go of. Their house was a refuge in a relationship perhaps beyond what society would consider 'normal'. As a pair they only visited Thornfield Court once. I tried to discus things sensibly but Danny ran off. I was probably jealous of him myself and he was only an eleven year-old boy! My neighbour downstairs was a black man named Frank and he brought Danny back up to flat 12 complaining the boy had been shouting and running about. The last time Sandy and I were on the air mattress together I felt extra need to 'perform' but fumbled the condom. I started crying. We never slept together again. The last evening I rode to Sandy's house I found no sign of life except for a light on in an upstairs window. I knocked on the door… and the light was switched off. It is likely that I myself had now become the threatening ex-boyfriend. Sandy had chosen her son over me. "Any mother would", I used to say. But I was bitter and, as is typical of the ends of most of my love affairs, I never saw her again.

Over two years before these events I made a synchronous link to Lord 'K' called the *Silver Shield*. Some of the co-incidences I communed through most people would have considered miraculous. *Silver Shield* was a name lifted from an insurance company yet I made the connection and it took on power that should be used with due care. I have had 'Kaos' communication before, found coherent statements flipping through a book that read as a satisfactory whole. So if you ever meet someone who claims there's no such thing 'co-incidence' be aware they maybe in the *Now*, in the *Between*, that they may see with their eyes much *more* than meets yours!

I used to worship in church, on Sundays, many deities at once. In the sitting room above the gas fire I made an altar. I placed two white candles on either end of the mantel and items that expressed higher forces in physical terms: a battery, a tea bag, a coin, perhaps a cross, some tobacco, a glass of water; maybe a couple of other things like a C.D. I became a *balancer*, the *Cabal*, the fifth in the midst of four – and many others. For over a week my opinions seemed respected and needed to stabilise the pros and cons of these forces. But the implication was that the *Cabal* position was un-winnable: the *"Hellbound Heart"* that (perhaps) can only be overcome by 'cheating'. But I was truthful; still am. I forged some modern views and encouraged some unexpected relationships and even walked away feeling pretty un-damned good about it! I wrote letters to my beloved Charlie Jordan often about what was happening. Thornfield Court was grim, but, like an occasionally missed target on a firing range, it was not always hurtful.

The place got in a mess but not nasty enough to be smelly. I cleaned it up before the community psychiatric nurse came to visit me. The C.P.N had been a part of my discharge arrangements with my consultant at The Lakes. The man I had been allocated was an old ex-prison officer. It was a vital exercise in 'pulling the wool' over his eyes to avoid hospital. Without television for the first few weeks, apart from sketching reaches, *Caballing*, and writing letters, I can't recall exactly how I spent the time; mostly speaking telepathically with the 'talk box' in my advanced brain. It went on and on continuously, but I did sleep – without *Zimmervane* – because the enemy wanted me to sling them out. I had a phone. I managed to get out a little, go dancing or visit Vagabonds café, and I used to buy C.D singles from a Sale in the main precinct, 1996 issues at £1 a throw. I used to play selections of them on Sunday mornings as a telepath DJ, or more accurately, as a DJ for telepaths. And of course I spoke to a genuine Radio One DJ, my special woman Charlie, in mirrors.

I was told the advanced brain runs on a magical chemical called Thoracic Cortisone. I enjoyed my other senses, the smell of roses and freshly washed clothes, the cool softness of my summer-time sleeping bag, and I started eating lunches in the garden by the honey-suckle tree. A law stated that I must eat fish rolls everyday, and that I must also have a fizzy drink with it, which I thought was to burp me to overcome sick-rapture. The method behind some of these attacks has since been forgotten in the intervening years. In one example, I saw a reddish visual of my shoes, or my bare feet, on the grass, while looking down at them *with my eyes shut*. In another I was in bed sometimes itching with what the enemy called 'mites'; they even made my skin itch if I was in a bath 'too long', making me jump out in a splash of water. Itching is why I've worn denim jeans almost everyday for over fifteen years! And why the cool cotton summer-time bag became so important. I rolled about a bit in bed, when going to sleep, movements that Barker called "the stations of the cross".

Outside my front door was a cement floor, downstairs, composed of tiles in patterns like large letter 'Y's. The upper landing was connected to the stairwell by a railing at the right angles, a balcony with a drop to the floor below of about twenty-seven feet. If you rolled off this backwards it would be as sure to kill you as a bullet in the head. So it became known as the "Y balcony", or just the 'Y', with at least two meanings. It could mean "Y *not* do?" as well as "Y do?"

Looking down at this structure gave me a feeling that fate had pre-arranged its terrible capability, like the window in my bathroom being embossed with boats and ships; a vision of the sea to assist against bladder-locks. I wrote about these things to Charlie. Perhaps I was proud of the indications of the forethought of higher forces. After splitting up with Sandy I wrote to Charlie of wanting another material (*vicinity one*) plane girlfriend to be with me. It wasn't to invoke jealousy it was because I needed physical comfort in that environment, where I was being hurt, sworn at, and threatened every day of the week. Promising Charlie that I would never go off the 'Y' seemed easy, then, but it would get worse later and I could never have known how bleak and terrible the situation would become.

CHAPTER THIRTEEN – JULY: 1997

I often postponed cleaning the flat with a sense of mild guilt. I didn't usually wash the dishes until the stuff was threatening to smash over the kitchen floor. When I did the job, finally, I had to contend with a terrible back-ache, when the enemy would say "He'll never do the washing up again." There were dirty clothes on the bedroom floor and although Mum wouldn't have minded washing them I rarely saw either of my parents. I had a life beyond them now. *High Acre* was a historical re-enactment, a museum of youth. Some telepath musicians encouraged me to clean the C.D.s and stack them respectfully on a table and I felt good afterwards. After the relegation of: *"You're not alone",* by Olive, my favourite song of this time was sung by Richard Ashcroft of *The Verve*. It was an emotive track with a beautiful violin melody entitled: *"Bitter Sweet Symphony".*

I purchased a VHS tape years before, distributed through the 'Redemption' label, of a pair of Barker's first B&W weirdo films called *"Salome"* and *"The Forbidden"*. I took them to the flat in West Mersea, watched them once and then the tape was accidentally exposed to an electric fan heater and melted! Barker had been writing his books during the most terrible years to me, 1997 and 1998. It had been business as usual for him. He had put the war-machine together long before and then let it rip. Before his Dog Company Theatre Company had met, Barker had built a team of men with varying evil specialities, I believed, enrolled to hurt me in allocated ways from when I was about four years old: brain mapping, biological manipulation, push-sub thoughts, 'nightmaring', and other capabilities with Barker himself as The Engineer. They have said I was never a child but that's bullshit. Based on some of my own memories I was a little boy that was tortured, needlessly so, most people would say, a tiny victim of sadism to mould me into the man they wished me to become.

In my journal, I wrote of my own dreadful circumstances and made diagrams from *reaches* that accounted global destiny and history. I drew the gargantuan *Incentimax* cylinder repeatedly, stacked with metaphorical Asgaroth / Deyaform constructions of galactic plates, thinking about a *Niagra*. I wrote 'tag' signs of the dominant participants in the conflict (the few that I knew about) and outlined my increasing suspicions of the *Helter Incendo*, of its motives, its raptures. I drew a circle of the Earth and another the same size, and sketched an arrow from the Earth to the second – the second, representing the *Helter Incendo*. I blocked in completely in black and started to get an inkling of danger on a planetary scale. I also drew a three by three, nine block map of how different *vicinities* connected and interrelated but I figured it was dangerous so I hid it in the cupboard with the telly!

One afternoon I felt the Earth tremble and believed that our atmosphere was being withdrawn by inter-dimensional 'gate' space ships, stripping our air with powerful vacuuming apparatus of unimaginable force. The souls were going up with an imminent *Niagra* into Quiddity – so I lay down and waited to die... someone shouted "hurry up!" but nothing happened. So about eight minutes later I got up and smoked a cigarette and had a cup of tea. Under an increasing mass of stress in the middle of the month I wanted to withdraw from the situation so I declared that I would never speak with telepathy again but it was to prove unmaintainable. You can't block out 'voices' by sticking your fingers in your ears, but I did get back on the horse... a recovery that became known as a 'bounce' (whimsically, the name of a brand of dog food!) When referring to the law that expressed the need to weep everyday, for fate, that month I just said "I'm not going to cry for the Earth anymore. I'm going to fight!" So I became a *Defender*.

Back in Lee and Jo's flat I had been challenged to take Charlie out of the *Helter Incendo*. Even with the enemy's suggestion of collecting three pomegranate seeds representing clues and methods, it remained a task I hadn't even the ghost of a vague idea of how to do. Even with a strong *imager* I couldn't simply visualise us out of the place.

It seemed the telepath *Dataform* net was rooted through Charlie's brain and when I was asked to make Law #100, I asked for: "a hundred more laws" and the entire list disappeared! I wrote to her everyday, love letters about what was happening, containing *maybes* and *possibles* and *aprox's* to adhere to the truth in the same way I'm recounting this memoir.

My *imager* was a vital tool, obviously. It was comprised of a gallows shaped *imagination drive* running through a diamond, a ruby and a sapphire. A crystal was stolen! The enemy must have known Charlie enjoyed the fun of opening and reading my letters, but writing them was trying because the monsters stepped up their attacks. The stolen crystal was used to refract new levels of pain while I was sitting on a bean-bag in the sitting room applying my pen. They assaulted me through ten new 'prismatic attack vicinities' a whirlwind of axes, whipping, shooting, nails, saws through spine, burning, and even my fundament lungs were ripped out of holes in my back and tied into an airless knot. Wanting the letters to be delivered on the same day, if I missed the last post I often rode down to the Royal Mail sorting office near the train station. Thankfully, my left wrist was strong enough to pull the clutch, and riding the bike somehow healed much of the agony that had been inflicted during writing.

I carried on as best I could: shaving, keeping clean, carrying the dirty washing to the laundrette on the back of my motorbike, and it was often painful. They said: "You're a masochist or else you would commit suicide". Yet not all my 'voices' were enemies. One of them rebuked them, saying: "a suicidal man wouldn't shave". And I developed another defence: nicotine. One cigarette to the next would keep me going at the worst times. While smoking I could 'attention grab' the places that hurt and apply it as an anaesthetic. "Increased grip" the enemy sometimes said when I lit up, or maybe it was "increased *grit*". There was no gemstone representing nicotine but I did learn about others. During a dream I remember grabbing back my own sapphire out of a CD box, before it snapped closed and when I woke up Barker said I had cheated. Being accused of 'cheating' indicated that I had done something right! Within three days, I found myself trying to hide another stone from all takers, a golden stone called The Bastion that sometimes spoke to me. So began a preoccupation of the time that I can't remember with complete clarity, but I do have the essence of it, which came to be called *The Crystal Frenzy*.

Stamp had *Rocks of Gore*, shining deep red, and stuck them into my fundament's chest. One caused a lot of agony, which thankfully eased until it disappeared. Barker had the *Stone of Yorin*, which had a connection with some dubious father, or other, of his. And in hospital I had learned that he was keeping something else 'close to his chest' – and *within* his chest – called the *'Heart box of Gordon'*. An inter-dimensional box full of crosses and six pointed stars representing the number of apocalyptic 'polices' he had arranged and the number of times he had killed me.

Charlie had a stone, too, the *Jordan Stone*, which she had found in her mind when she had been little.
I was awarded a special white diamond called *The Global Peace Music Bastion* that may have improved my appreciation of music but it was stolen by Toni Braxton! I discovered a podium that was like a traditional cake stand in my mind on which I could keep my collection out of reach of grasping *scu* hands but stones and gems were begged, borrowed, and stolen all the time. Custody changed so often we started stashing our crystals in our own personal Mandlebroth Sets: repeating Kaos like bottomless safe deposit boxes with only one genuine gem in an endless column of identical fakes. Barker's stone wasn't long or sharp enough for him. So one night while I was lying on the air-mattress he stuck a thing called a *Yorin Spar* straight through my chest. It all ended after my stone and Charlie's *Jordan Stone* hid together behind a wooden cross, hanging outside the kitchen. Their progeny may have too glamorous

to cope with. The *Frenzy* was calmed and the *Crystals* became valueless. It had been a tiring challenge, but fun, in its way.

I had been writing letters to Charlie Jordan now and then for one hundred and sixty weeks. I never had a reply. I didn't even have a photograph. It was frustrating, and I tried to keep a lid on the discontent but I believed it was because I was a no one in the world of entertainment. The job in London was an ancient position; by 1997 I had no contacts, no contracts, no representation and a C.V riddled with a pox of redundancy and mental illness. I deeply loved her, and I knew that if there was <u>firm contact</u> between us the war might end, but the enemy made it quite clear: "He's Joe," they used to say, "He's Joe", meaning I was '*Joe Public*'. I was locked out.

I wanted letters, and not only from Charlie. I wanted the recognition of telepath celebrities. Whether signed or not, and however secretive, in their perspective such contact could cause an unimaginable disaster. In spite of the adage 'never make an oath' I swore I wouldn't show the letters to anyone – especially not to the psychiatric industry. This was a vow I would have kept. Envelopes hidden in the wardrobe? Tied with a thin red ribbon? They would have been no one else's verifier but mine. Then came a chance for me to 'pick the lock': The BBC was coming to East Anglia! Radio One were going to hold a summer road-show twenty miles from Colchester. The whole kit was being staged in Clacton-on-sea on 5th August, near the beach on the Marine Parade (West) and I knew it could be the perfect opportunity to meet Charlie. There was a bar called *Tom Peppers* down the road and I posted her instructions to meet me there after the show. Because of the essentially faceless nature of a radio personality I tried to assure her that she wouldn't be recognised. As far as I knew no visual promotion had ever been made of Charlie. I had been trying to get her photograph on and off for years! Yet I thought she would appear lovely to me when we met, smiling face to face, sensually mouth to mouth; a situation of amazing possibilities!

So early that morning of 5th August, I dressed in black motorcycle leathers and rode off with a frame of mind like the fear clamped upon before a parachute jump. That is an exaggerated metaphor but I was excited indeed. The sun was shining, and in places the Clacton Road is a superb ride. As I've said to other people before, the corners have some satisfying sweeping curves. I parked the machine up a few minutes from the town centre, locked the ignition, and on my way through I bought a sweet dark rose from a florist. The show couldn't have been missed and neither could I because I sat like a sore thumb right in midst of a crowd of about fifty kids! D.J Lisa I. Anson waved at me, which was nice – that's what I believed at the time.

I had the sensation of a huge telepathic kiss. It was like leaving an air-conditioned aeroplane, walking into the exit and being blanketed with humidity. A kiss of love, projected from the lead singer of a band called *Casino*. In spite of a slipped thought that the band might have been named by Barker, and therefore a trap, I was enjoying the event. It was going down like a pina colada in the Caribbean! Jimmy Sommerville, who I thought was a woman when I first heard him, sang his latest song. But it was when people were filtering away *after* the show that my time was coming. In the merchandising trailer I asked if Charlie 'was around the back' and the worker said she didn't know. While I walked to Tom Peppers I saw a red 'people-mover' with Lisa I. Anson and a few other passengers driving away from the site but I didn't think Charlie was in it.

The bar smelt of beer and cigarette smoke. It was dim and busy as a fun-fair exhibit. She would be afraid of public drunks but I found a table free with two chairs waiting in the semi-detached intimacy of a bay window at the front. Tourists milled about, to and fro in the sun, oblivious to this potentially historic moment. I slipped Charlie's rose into a glass of water, or maybe it was a bottle. I was *less sure* she would meet me than my *certainty* that she was in Clacton... I sat there trying to push the possibility of failure away like it was a wooden bar feebly holding back crashing disappointment. My controlled suppression of this fear was channelled into a countdown – after we would split up.I had tried my best, yes, but wasn't I also transferring the remainder of my inadequacy into Charlie's responsibility? At zero we would be done with in as many essences of 'zero' as you can think of.

A telepath was doing the counting, a mystery man who was being unnecessarily hard but I didn't realise that the countdown was really *for me*. And soon it was done. I was left as stranded and as partnerless and alone as ever.

The *Helter Incendo* was growing. My fundament was carried nightly into its depths where I was cut open. My jewelled *Heart Box of Glory* was lifted out and replaced with a rusty container of frogs of living shit called a *Stamp Box*. Before they shut the lid one of them may have urinated in it with piss that stung like acid. But I found an answer. I blotted up the pain, and the heat, the itching, until I jumped out of bed in a state of broken distraction to run a bath and fetch an apple from the fridge. While having a soak I ate the cool green fruit and felt much better; clean, tired. Connected to the Garden of Eden story I was given thirty minutes of healing, assisted by the forbidden force apples represent – *The Art,* and then got to sleep. But there were testing dreams.

Stamp called his nightmares 'Happy Times' compiled on *Tapes 1 - 4*. Being able to have an influence over these bloody scenes he called "considerate" – and, inversely, being driven by force and having no choices Stamp, not surprisingly, called "inconsiderate". Some of the dreams were for the disgust of telepaths only, a campaign of toilet horror that I don't think I ever dreamt myself. One morning I woke up and was told I had kicked Howard Stern, an associate of Barker's, to death: jumped on his head in the semi-lucid dream-level called *Agro form*. But I don't remember that either. I walked out miraculously unscathed from others, such as reaching the outskirts of a nightmare Stamp had called "Doom" and some were so terrible I've been told I curled up and actually went to sleep *within the dream!*

I recalled 1997 as being adventurous, a description I obviously didn't apply at the time. I discovered an interior vicinity called the *Universe Generator* made of a metal akin to 'copper', perhaps the ghost of a suit of armour I had worn into ancient battles. It might also have been an enemy battle-platform. On one Sunday afternoon, listening to the Radio One Top 40 show while smoking a Marlboro, a seductive space had emanated from me. It was an essence of pure relaxation, deep blue and glittering with golden stars. S*cu* observed the wonder of it from a balcony rail yet the 'Qualm' Air-Gate Commander *Peloquin* had suddenly sucked the *Generator* until it was empty – and then smacked his lips as if appreciating a particularly fine bottle of cold beer! Another time, *Peloquin* had sucked up the pleasant holiness emerging from Canterbury Cathedral as I walked towards it. I gathered he was storing up these essences in his legs to share with his wife 'after'.

The oceanic space I had generated then may have inspired my artistic instinct. I bought a block of twelve A2 blank cards and some brushes and Acrylic paints. I placed the card on a baseboard perched on a pile of bean bags and applied washes of colour with a window behind me, painted blue 'vortexes' with pink features of hearts and balloons and bells and teardrops illuminated by the light shining over my shoulders. The enemy had to counter my initiative. They used push–subs called *style rapture*, a hypercritical fussy perception of manipulated disappointment but it backed-fired on them because although Acrylic paint does dry quickly it forced me into a state of near perfectionism. The pink features contrasted out of the surrounding blue with a couple of lovers kissing and cuddling in each, sometimes surrounded in a blue so dark it was almost black, with a shimmering crystal in each.

I also tapped in tiny white stars, with my '0000' brush, directed by a tiny 'attention grab' forming them into constellations. I painted nine pictures in all, all close to perfect. The other 'vortexes' that followed were not up to the same standard. I stopped painting.

That bedtime feeling of being small and cuddled up in a duvet without fear of pain was targeted. I was hounded about the night sedation I had saved up 'because it was a drug' and the bottle rattled
when I threw it in the bin. The enemy continued to manipulate my body temperature, "had me hot", in the colloquial parlance, and sometimes they did this by burning my *fundament* body. Without the summer-time bag I would have tossed and turned, and Ellison hunted for a 'closed eye view', trying to get me to hallucinate with my eyes shut in the black of night. It was a hijacked *imager*, not *intenseiform* but dark strings grew over my inner eye and they never beat it. Without the *Zimmervane* I often felt more awake trying to get to sleep than when I was trying to wake up!

After leaving Sandy I had been going out to bars, clubs, and Vagabonds Café to meet young women since July. Having been rail-roaded at the road-show I left Tom Peppers and went hunting 'talent' but I was inept. I could make the initial approach but I always fumbled the balls because I had no sense of humour. A couple of times in a pub I had a few laughs with 'goth' people clad in black clothing with piercings and stainless steel jewellery, after a thing called a 'bone of hue' had been meshed with my body. It was in my chest. It made everything comical but there is never a 'bone of hue' around when you really need one. Basically girls love funny stuff and I had none. Facing a pretty new face I was scorched by her gaze and ended up like a watering hole, always drying up and retreating! The more beautiful she appeared the more difficult it was to dredge up conversation and nothing was helped by the enemy's bullshit 'advice'. I continuously believed all they said, my understanding perhaps both literally and metaphorically not my own.

The chance of 'pulling', so they said, is more likely if the girls are in groups of odd numbers. They said I would be in more danger if I looked into a man's vulnerable left eye, especially if he was drunk, because the 'shielding' on most people's right eyes bump together harmlessly. Of the dominance of women in groups, they said that the lower females stayed near their more charismatic 'alpha female' to jealously keep others away, particularly courting men. These tactics generated caustic complications. They said people were upset by the scars on my left wrist. They said every decent looking woman was already seeing someone who I would have to fight. As I've said before

I avoid fighting because after a life-time of manipulated fear, and hate of adrenaline, hate even of the *possibility* of adrenaline, my 'normal' fight-or-flight instincts may have been disturbed. I don't like being hit and I certainly don't at all like hurting anybody else.

Colchester is Britain's oldest recorded town. Set back from where Queen Street joins the round-about at the bottom are some ancient ruins: Creamy bright roofless walls in the sunlight; arches and tombs on the soft grass – all that remains of St. Botolph's Priory. Summer can see a gathering place there for drunks and drug users. I was lying on my back listening to a cassette of Beethoven on a second hand pocket stereo (that was new to me) and someone was standing over me. The man was talking. He looked rough so I plucked out my earphones and learned he wanted to borrow my Walkman because his girlfriend had died recently and he wanted to listen to their favourite song. So I lent it to him. He took the machine back to his friends as pleased as a magpie with a shiny bottle top.

The third time I went back to try to retrieve it, three of them came after me. I might have managed to get in one punch and a kick as I ran, but I scraped my bare left arm on a ruined wall and had to curl up in the defensive fetal position. I took a few kicks, which didn't seem to hurt, until I finally

172

shouted "ALRIGHT!" and they stopped. That split second of rage has happened to me before. Leaving the scene I met a tall vagrant wearing a large red cross who I thought was a 'street policeman'. I did not ask for his assistance because I didn't want enemies around town, capable of such violence, to remember me, and I also ignored a genuine law officer. I walked to The Three Crowns pub nearby and, with a few post trauma tears, washed the blood off the scrape to my arm in the toilet saying: "I've had a hard day at the office" in the mirror. Within an hour I was asking to test a £55 Sony Walkman and when the staff's back was turned I walked out of the shop with it clamped in my hands like a steering wheel. There were no security guards, nor store detectives, no comebacks of any kind. I had replaced the machine I had lost at the ruins – with a brand new one!

Vagabonds café was where I made strong friendships that I still value today. I also met a beautiful woman named Rowen. She was well spoken with an Earth mother's body and dark flowing hair,
a "chip off the old block" of Ruth Ann Regan, vocalist of the band *All About Eve*. She had a proud back and worked in a branch of *Waterstones Books*. The pages of my journal began to feature her with increasing eroticism, and the hope that we might see each other. I had to contend with an added *scu* manufactured terror when I walked into her shop. Making an unusual bid for her attention I laid a paper-chase with clues hidden in books that featured a cartoon of Rowen as a squirrel rushing around on a skate-board. The last one I hid was an invitation to the café for a tall glass of iced mango tea. I was stood up. She must have crumpled up the first clue, or not received it from the colleague of hers that I had asked to pass it on… whatever the reason I was going to have to accept, soon, that she simply didn't fancy me.

She had clique of associates and friends in Colchester that were unseen but which surrounded her like a fortress. I almost fought one of them outside Vagabonds. I wanted to smack him on the head with a stick of French bread but I just couldn't do it. While I was out on the town she sent me away

173

when I sat near her. She avoided my eyes, and avoided me in the café. Seeing that I didn't want to be a stalker I decided that she was a lost cause... or was it *me* that was becoming a lost cause...to myself?

Around that last week, of August '97, I had an experience both pleasing and strange: I took on the outlook and personality of a woman! I felt fully 'contained' within my own body, and it was so comfortable I had thought that it was some kind of reward from Barker, or his side-kick Ellison!
I bought white 'T' shirts from women's rails in charity shops, with labels like *Dorothy Perkins*, and I came across a few raptures for women – like that the time 11:45 am makes some housewives feel tired and need a rest. I wandered around the flat once or twice feeling like I was pregnant! There was virtually no fighting to be done at the end of that month, a time when the enemy experimented in control. They most likely used the *scu* of a woman on a full brain lock – *'possession'* in other words – and it was a highly sensual experience however short lived. Inevitably the action of August went back into history, so I went back into making history as a man of action.

In the absence of Charlie Jordan I was introduced to telepath women. Ruth Anne Regan described herself as "horror". I couldn't believe *All About Eve* was a beautiful 'front' for some kind of demon. Or the possibility I suppressed that Ruth Anne had taken the mantle of evil because she thought that being lovely and playing happy folk music was boring. The actress Holly Hunter manifested beside me in my bedroom but her face was horribly twisted by *The Art*. The only woman that the enemy actually *allowed* me to court was Olive, because the word NOT also meant the almost unimaginable end of the soul. I went clubbing with Olive's image. She was cheeky and funny. That September I went to London to meet her at the National Gallery. I came across a 30-something year old woman in there wearing spidery black stockings but she said she wasn't Olive. It was like Ireland again, like Clacton. Trying to work out a bonus from this disaster I shoplifted a poster from the shop and walked to the exit, without metal shutters coming down, or klaxons, or security guards, while thinking: "Wow, I'm stealing a painting from the National Gallery!!"

The total of *Natural* women I approached between mid July and mid September numbered over one hundred and forty. I didn't forge a relationship. I encouraged a girl to whom I was close to borrow my journal, which I believed it was a life-changing read, but she knew Rowen and after she handed it back to me I don't think I saw her again. The two or three telephone numbers I had collected resulted in flashes of interest that burnt cold, and all of this was bringing me back to Charlie. If it wasn't for my letters, her imitator (that I had gathered was Sharlene Spiterie) would have deafened Charlie and I to each other. Later in the conflict that is exactly what happened. One day I had contact with my loved one for less than two seconds.

You don't appreciate something until it's gone and in this example I mean physically: mind voice, imagination, smell, visual memory – all were destroyed by October. My sinuses were stunned by *rapture* so the pleasantness of freshly laundered clothes, one of my favourite smells, had no scent. I could enjoy a rose only by pushing my nose deep into its petals. The block of 360 random access slides of my imagination, which used to be so vaulted and full of colours while I was reading, was stripped out. I could project an image forward over-laying Material Plane *(vicinity one)* reality but the "motion picture reading system" went one slide at a time during attacks that even I considered impossible. Yet it happened. The enemy used alternative visualising 'screens' (except perhaps for their own forward projection) but the imagination behind my own thoughts has since been dim.

I hope not, but when I start to write new fiction it might be like trying to drive a car on four flats! My memory-board was also deconstructed into still-frames with a low factual accuracy sometimes confused with manufactured images. I was happy about the way people admired my mind voice. They said it was pleasant, and it was pleasing to use so for that the enemy raptured my *talk-box* down into the cavity at the roof of my mouth, and placed a six legged 'eater machine' in there. It was made of shiny metal that crunched and scratched the flesh. Trying to 'talk' with that was like trying to communicate through broken glass, so I had to talk aloud. It disturbed Frank and my other neighbour downstairs, Andrew, but I only recall one complaint from them in many months. Mum visited me sometimes with a box of provisions and a worried smile, but my parents weren't a part of my world.

Once again in the kitchen I was in much pain stooping over the washing up. Harvey Kietel was shooting me in the spine with a gun that fired dry tomatoes. It was quite painful. I heard Harvey represented tomatoes (perhaps with a capital 'T') and his weapon might have made a highly original multi-dimensional gun in a film, perhaps directed by one of his friends? How about a gun that shoots a variation of other vicious dried fruit and vegetables? Every morning I smoked and had a cup of tea for breakfast. At night I often cooked dinners usually using only four weird ingredients like old bread and mustard mayonnaise. Every time I cooked Stamp said he'd kill himself if I ate it on a bed of lettuce. There is never any lettuce around when you need it.

Back in May *'intonsiforming'* into Stamp's ziggurat temple proved to be nothing to worry about. I never really took it seriously. I actually thought *'intonsiforming'* was a silly word and re-defined it to mean flipping over three hundred and sixty degrees, with some imagination, back into a sitting position. It raised a smile. If someone felt happy they would suddenly say: "I'm intonsiforming," and back-flip! Maybe I did poke fun at Stamp then, but I had witnessed his vileness. The *scu* of Alannis Morrisette visited me once and told me that her woman had been terribly upset at seeing a fly in her soup. I became tearful because I thought it had been Stamp's *intenseiform* but in fact it had been a real fly. People used to say "in-tennis-form" to calm Stamp down, and he usually used the term *'intenseiform'* as a general word applying to all of his attacks. The creaking noises of the building settling at night, one click for "yes" and two clicks for "no", I believed had been Godly communication. Stamp insisted he was doing it and he said the word *'intenseiform'* with a grim and dark pronunciation, but I had forgotten he lied all the time anyway.

Spending too much time alone with a mental illness I now consider dangerous. You are never truly alone with 'voices' so I kept pets. I purchased a large bird-cage and a cockatiel, and back in July I bought a small hamster, a little grey Russian with beady eyes and twitching whiskers. When I was taking him out of his box he bit me and I wept. Soon he escaped from my unfriendly wooden version of a hamster box and had the freedom of the floor. I left saucers of food and water out for him. Since he used to disappear for two or three days at a time and return looking exactly the same I called him 'Tardis'. I was brewing tea in the kitchen one day and I looked at the untouched plate of hamster seed in the corner of the floor that I had placed there beside a hole in the kitchen units three days ago. And when I glanced back at it a moment later, a third of the food had vanished and there – looking identical to how he had appeared when he left – was Tardis!

Like the describable differences between Barker and myself, which the artist had outlined personally, I was told Charlie Jordan was represented by a dog and that Sharlene Spiterie was represented by a horse. Charlie was a King Charles Cocker Spaniel, like *'Lady'* in the Disney animation: *"The Lady and The Tramp"* and Sharlene was a pale mare. I kept a small dog of that breed myself but that winter is sadly bereft of memories of her. I was too ill to live comfortably with the dog until 1998. I wanted to call her 'Charlie' or 'Charlotte' but her first owner had named her 'Lottie'. I kept the name. It is an old lady's name for Charlotte anyway.

Once I accepted I couldn't name my cockatiel after my loved one because he was male, the bird was the truest joy to me. He was a beautiful young example with pale blue and green plumage and the stance of a falcon. He had a quill of feathers on top of his head that flattened when he was scared and stood up when he was happy and sometimes he squawked! He strutted up and down his wooden bar tentatively, like the way he pecked his seed, and I put his house on the low table beside my bed. I talked to him about the day's news, gradually earning his trust, and called him Beaky Bird. While he was sleeping I draped a towel over his

house so that he wouldn't be disturbed by the early morning light, or the candle I burned every night. Soon I was able to coax him onto my index finger, his little talons gripping firmly, and then he had full air-space of the flat. I left birdseed near the ceiling in the lounge up-lighter and, somehow, water. I walked about with Beaky standing on my head, and lifted my finger to kiss him, but that is my last strong memory of the bird. One day I returned to the flat and he was gone. I never knew the circumstances.

Each white church candle was an icon that was usually shoplifted. I burned one every night, a beacon that became known as the *'Candle of Hope'*. Enemy raptures were continuous and often combined. At night I started to feel a phantom gun in my dominant hand while sleeping. In some mirror trapped corner of my vision was a puppet of Barker flapping its eyes at me, which I thought was funny. The essence of the hand pistol I clutched was designed to engineer you to purchase a firearm within six weeks. So in London I bought a small white New Testament Bible and I held that in my hand instead. The rapture faded. This technique may actively encourage sleep and has since been updated to holding a "hand-cuddler" in your hand, such as a squashy cat. Ellison said: "there is no such thing as a hand-cuddle" but why not go shopping for a soft toy, or doll, like you loved when you were little? The "Batty eyed Clive" puppet was terrible. It was difficult to get rid of and designed to change one's sexual orientation. Make a heterosexual man gay.

I hadn't 'sensually relieved' myself for several days (I had no naughty books and my imagination had been destroyed) and my desire for women was disappearing into a chasm of men's nuts and bolts. One night it all came to a head, if you'll pardon the pun, when I was *push-subbed* into a state of ruination through the hideous batty eyed puppet and an offensive image of a singer who's music had been imprinted on me when I was a teenager, music that for me had the atmosphere of innocent `and happy love affairs. All connection to that naivety was punched with holes when I hallucinated this favoured singer handling his disgusting erect penis. Full of horror I suddenly snapped. I ran into the bathroom and collapsed on the floor with the lights out, hollowed and rolling around screaming. Later I went back to my bedroom. I sat on the air-mattress and I was rescued… words filed passed me outside the window about others in my spiritual family; Beauty, Joy, Happiness. It was special, and lovely, and comforting; I drifted off in my summer-time bag, with 'Fred'.

I believed I had been victorious over the gun rapture but I bought an air pistol. It cost me about seventy pounds despite the fact that I didn't often have any money. As a veteran gambler since about the age of ten I was attracted to the tactile mystery of slots that screwed me, more than once, out of every coin I had; and the bus fare home. I have felt relief walking out of an 'amusement' arcade back onto the street with no money left because it meant I had no money left to gamble with. So powerful was this addiction it caused me to commit crimes, but I learned that my fingers hadn't been the only influence over those buttons. I had been enslaved by a Barker's *deep set programme #16*, and it had cost thousands.

A *deep set programme* was a manipulation applied in clusters to the advanced brain, a weapon to generate rising sub-thoughts that can drive a telepath to deeds it's not likely they would have done if they'd been left alone. Many *deep programmes* had been pasted in a long time ago, anticipatory and pertinent to modern war. Some emphasised the pros and cons of names. Others were more detailed, with phrases that indicated a grasp of psychology:
"Never post Richard-Clement-with-the-'es', a letter." Or "You love Charlie Jordan more than Richard" Or "You will pew with sick quickly if you see Charlie and Richard together in a public place". And we also discovered *power-words*, Barker's groundwork for a masquerade of fake thoughts – for the creation of his allies and the embryos of my future enemies. It was uncovered in mid-September using Charlie Jordan's own tactic of crumpling sheets of imaginary newspaper rising to the top of your head, with legible pages of *deep programmes* rising with them. Unearthed, assessed, the situation faded to memory.

The girl next door was in her early 20's and worked for the Post Office. I visited once, her living-room hippy with pastel colours. She had been using hashish at the time. Even passively smoking it made me feel like my brain was swelling and I went back to Flat 12 where the enemy accused me of sampling it. I denied that but I felt a long needle being pushed into my brain that punctured my pituitary gland, like one of the mad L.S.D 'marples' of 1991. They sucked up the secretion with it and said it was the 'elixir of life'. I never went back to her flat again for any significant length of time. Many similar attacks above the shoulders have also defied logical explanation. I wandered around Flat 12 once with the sensation of creatures crawling through my brain called 'Stern Worms'. They were fed into the ear of my *fundament* and they truly felt like slippery worms. If I'd heard the name Howard Stern before '97 I had forgotten it. After smoking a cigarette or drinking tea, or coffee, another problem could occur. The awareness of 'brain-taste', which was easy for a *scu* to alter the flavour to the likes of a 'sulphur bomb' that twice reduced my thought processes into a dust bowl.

'Addiction' was becoming accusatory. The nature of smoking was brought up several hundred times, mostly because it assisted me. I could have called them anaesthetics, but you can die of too much anaesthetic, also. *Scu,* and perhaps the odd soul, sampled inter-dimensional cigarettes *(feelie-sticks)* and took cups of caffeinated drinks from The Drive-Bar, a shrunken down place at the back of my head. Inter-vicinity manipulation of size, by force of will, has at least two verbs: shrinkage is known as a *brick-down*, and enlarging yourself bigger maybe called a *brick-through*. The drinks were also highly addictive to subtle bodies, more so than in the example of physical people, but you try going without coffee or tea for a month – you'd be climbing the fucking walls! The enemy said 'cigarette'. I said: "Burn the sticks but don't let *them* burn *you!*"

My information was that *subtle bodies* had to die 2000 times to get out of the *Helter Incendo*. It was still growing, and it was composed of *Dimension Two*. I didn't know what this material was composed of but I had learned that the place was terrible, particularly to *feelies*. That was why the inhabitants were mostly *scu*, maybe some *fundaments*. That month I was separated from the busy side of that vicinity by a river the enemy that couldn't cross, so I was alone and safe. But I was itching to attack. I had been tricked into saying I wouldn't attack with music, but that month, armed with a barrage of hard-core trance, I crossed the river with images of red spheres solidifying through my limited visualiser, called 'orbital lasers'. I fired them left and right, and felt shivers from the dark bass-line in the thrill of the assault that sometimes made my skin feel like it was breaking into goose bumps. Once I flew three blasting away at the same time, but it was a spectacular waste of effort. The enemy just mended the damage instantaneously using a defence called *memory-return*. The mass of shattered material was rejuvenated by their 'time-turning' of memory made solid, resetting the place to the condition it had been in *before* the attack had happened. But it was when I had grasped the essence of *'brick-through'* that I really had them on the run.

The size of my 5'11" physical body was approximately 144 times bigger than the *scu* in the *Incendo* when I meshed the place with a telephone directory on the carpet. Sliding the book aside, with my thumb about twice their size, I squashed them with it. I could see the tiny little enemies in the broad light of day and chose my targets instinctively. I picked out many because they started running for the exits at the back. *Memory return* must have been tiresome because they began dividing the floors. They hid at least two levels, one under the next, in layers I found difficult to penetrate.

Thornfield Court became combined with the *Helter Incendo* on a 1:1 scale initially in four places. My bedroom and lounge had a control room *bricked down* in the wall in between them, and that was inhabited by the Air-Gate Commander *Peloquin* and a man we shall call *The Editor*. The cupboard by the front door had an elevator in it that led down into Stamp's area, because his nick-name was Frank and that was also the name of my neighbour downstairs, but this area never did feature in any situation. In a corner, by the wardrobe away from the bottom of my air-mattress, was a door that led onto Barker's balcony. It overlooked an auditorium that was evidence of how gigantic the vicinity had become. The arena could hold thousands. His door also 'conveniently' opened onto my bedroom. My toilet was meshed with another called the "pew the goo seat", to induce perversion. The 'social area' was attached to the far corner of my living-room along a corridor that, because I didn't know what was underneath it, I assumed was an aerial walkway. This was the *Helter Incendo*, also known as *Vicinity Two*. It was a trap fattening itself on people's misery and still maturing.

I learned it might have existed in Barker's brain also. Through our link he was trying to transfer it to mine like an ambassador shredding documents before evacuating a crisis. My own notes almost caused a 'document frenzy' until I posted them to 'significant others' at an address long forgotten. I couldn't control a *scu* of my own, except perhaps a *dream scu*. My actions and decisions were watched by the JUD. This meant: "Jordan You Deliver" but even if they had been *real* judges I never showed them much new. Regarding truth, I felt I could not lie. I still had no idea of how to get Charlie out of there but be that as it may I believed the members of the JUD had been hand picked by the enemy in the first instance. The *Helter Incendo* was as black as Barker's heart and as dark as the evenings passing earlier into autumn. Its depths were as concealed and as secretive as telepathy itself and it sometimes seemed so huge I felt helpless. So I set up my television set, in the living-room. I had a suspicion that this was going to be a very long winter.

'Life' in Thornfield Court had the essence of underlying expectation that was like having
your mind ready on the buttons of a pin-ball game, an anticipation evolving too slowly to
be noticed. Logic can be defied by tactility. Can a simulation *felt physically* actually <u>be</u> a 'simulation'? How can independent personalities seize such control over your body? The 'burden of truth' generated by these questions is a falsehood. It is schizophrenia, and when it is healed, you can look back upon those days as a dark dream and you'll have loads of time because you survived. Then you can truly live. Brighter dreams: of driving a car or making a home, dreams of a normal life, can be realised.

I loved dreaming. I annotated them onto lengths cut from art-paper that I called a 'Night Strip', wrote them by the light of the *Candle of Hope*. Its flame could be seen as far away as London, as a piercing blue beacon in the distant darkness. Reading Night Strips the next day brought back a little of the scenery of those adventures, but I suppose I liked it too much because the faculty was wiped out. I was known to say "even a nightmare is better than no dream at all" but that depends on what the nightmare is made of. Within a few minutes of my going to sleep the *scu* assembled in front of 'the dream screen' in the *Helter Incendo* to witness a fakery of false images that were not mine. Toilet horrors were projected. Barker would say "ah… a toil" but when I learned my reputation was being exposed to this sewage I *pretended* to sleep. Then I would set the screen on fire: raze it to the ground because another power in this war was rooted in what people believe – and belief *en-mass* can tear down castles of the blackest stone.

I wasn't eating properly and I felt like I was being worn down like a soft pencil. Most days for a little while, I sat at my table to write to Charlie. One day I scribbled something randomly, like art meshed with another's signature, and suddenly I felt inter-dimensional muck begin pouring invisibly out of my mouth! I scribbled another and a torrent of 'nusifiers', or *dimension two*, forced apart my jaws as it gushed out until my teeth gradually closed back together. And I found others. It was an amazing discovery of subliminal messages with different functions from first-draft scribbles. They became known as *sublims,* which could induce: rapture defence / attack; dumping matter-collectors; sleeping assistance, happy feelings, and perhaps interior vicinity 'cleaning'. I sent packets of them to Charlie.

The enemy said that I'd "had it planned!" and indeed it could have been an arrangement made before we were born. Celebrities in the L. A. vicinity told me that possibly their *feelie souls* had been raptured into insects, so I went up against Barker himself and applied a sublim that ejected the insect-form and cleansed them of their difficulties, but it may have been a simulation. My belief in all their bullshit was my worst problem. Lies like poisoned weeds strangled my sanity. My 'voices' manufactured realities truer to me than the world of everybody else and called them *vave-simulations*. I was told 'Vave' was the old word for 'pain' and I lapped up all this apocrypha like a thirsty animal. "Worlds within worlds" as Barker himself has written, and what they were saying to me sounded so *true*. Some folks shouted "Stop belief!" which was good advice that in my left hand heart I understood perfectly well but buried it there. Then in the blind spot in the corner of my dominant right eye I discovered the source that was exaggerating the essence of Barker's lies: the *swit*.

It looked like a red circle, a clock but with one hand and no numbers. Telepathy sounded as neutral as anyone else's when the hand pointed due north; at north-east it sounded very 'true' and north-west like 'lies' – all felt deep within one's instincts like the rising sub-thought of a *deep-set programme*. I had somehow been a 'telepathy routing-point' since childhood. Barker had been operating the *swit* through my neural nets, somehow interfacing the device with my own brain about twenty-seven years ago. He had hidden behind its capability ever since. I always adapted quickly to problems and I was pleased Barker had been caught in the blind spot behind the bike sheds attacking people's tires with a failed rapture coin that had his head on both sides! He may have been addicted to the power of it, sold *swits* for cash dollars saying it was "a legitimate weapon for this time of year." While on the subject of apocalypse I heard that the *swit* is made of the same material as the *Helter Incendo* – the dark suspicious mystery of *Dimension Two*. Barker offered me one of my own, in a bid to keep his. I said "No".

Vave-simulation was starkly real to me, situations measured by role-playing enemies. The action was seamless and I cued the consequences in these unfolding plots. Many friendships were wrecked by simulation. I drifted apart from long favoured Artists because of things that never happened. They may not have even known what crimes they were supposed to have done and probably wondered how the hell I could believe any of it. I ate less and fought more.
I sometimes stirred the cold ashes of those burnt-out friendships but the damage was done.

Some vave-sim challenges were based on my own *Reacher,* about proportion, about the macro-cosm *bricked down* into the micro-cosm; about infinity in a circle and a universe in a sphere the size of an egg. Perhaps second only to a thing I had with the Time Lords, my interaction with the *Cusper Plane* was consistently front-stage. It was deadly game that continued for so long that the role-players may have stopped playing. It became an adventurous reality to them also. My opinions, like an affective award nomination, produced rank-and-file Cuspers including Peloquin himself: a hierarchical army of Air-Qualm and Water-Qualm, (*feelies* and aliens, both) that I saluted in mirrors. But they were in Barker's back pocket box and they had the dreadful power to control our re-incarnation.

Like banging my head on a kitchen unit, I got so angry once I attacked the door to the boiler-cupboard with a screw-driver. I stuck it into the wood four times then hallucinated a dribble of blood from the last hole that was not my image. It took the wind out of me. Within three minutes I had taken the door off the cupboard and carried it down to the trash dumping room. I was highly-strung but I enjoyed "going soft"; R & R wrapped in a duvet and a sleeping bag. I had 'Fred', and I watched television by the warmth of the gas fire. I felt small and happy.

Listening to music can also enhance relaxation and an experience millions have in common is listening to music while they are sleep. I believed hearing music during slumber can induce deeper colours of REM. At school in Langley Park, I loaded my stereo with relaxing soul by Sade, when going to bed, because I had heard it from another room and it seemed like an adult thing to do. But the more desperate you are for something the less likely you are to get it. I couldn't reach even the first dream-level and had to switch the machine off.

In Canterbury cathedral I believed that a high up God wanted to sleep to its ambient sounds, to sleep on the cool rock under that huge vaulted ceiling to the choir. So I curled up in a corner but I couldn't reach sleep and I was soon told to "move along". I've been denied music-sleep by the enemy for as long as I have been listening, since *Level 42* and *Gary Numan*, and the time could be described like a prison term: "Fifteen years to Life" without intentional music-sleep yet it wasn't important to me until I was twenty-eight. One night in flat 12 I was playing a compilation of relaxing chill-out, called *Café del Mar: Volume One*, and I actually slept! I had been out for only a few minutes, to track #8, but I jumped awake feeling refreshed. The achievement would have a huge bearing on events later that winter.

In Barker's novel *The Great and Secret Show* the mortal enemies of the Earth were waiting to cross the Dream Sea to conquer us. That looked like "mountains of fleas" because they were composed of miniscule 'spore' called *lad*

Oroboros. At one point I had considered the possibility that Barker was an *lad agent*, that he had secreted them in an interior vicinity in his legs represented by a dreadful 'tag' signature that looked like a high voltage electricity warning. There were other 'spore' known as *ratnika* that could damage flesh and bone and enamel, and both were deployed against me that October. I needed a dentist because I've had *ratnika* in my teeth since I was eleven. These spores were left within me to fight it out and not even Peloquin wanted anything to do with them. He just attended closely, sucking his extra strong mentholyptus, and anticipating any genuinely precious essence.

An emergency *scu*-quarantine was declared. *lad* liked warmth and sweetness like chocolate: and they could kill a soul; *Ratnika* preferred coolness, particularly liked the cans of cold Stella Artois I drank of an evening to assist sleep. They were at odds with each other, while I laid on the air-mattress – fought in my blood stream like my body was a long tray made up of 'electrified ball bearings in hot oil' that swayed with the tilt and yaw of bedtime. I was stuffed with these balls that bumped about randomly in what children at school learn is called 'Brownian Motion'. I was visited by the writer Tom Sharpe and the singer Carol Decker of *T'Pau*. The gist of it was that eons ago, when their spores had been cancelled by suicide, they had been thus rewarded. Their visit had most likely been a *vave-sim* used to destroy friendships or to aid in destroying me.

Charlie or Sharlene told me that the *lad* had an appetite for mayonnaise, so I off-loaded some into a jar of Helman's, and was told their munching would turn some of the cream yellow. I enjoyed the unequivocal evidence! Since the *lad* could move along television lines they could therefore travel in time as well as geographically. It upset my 'going soft'. That people's souls could be destroyed by watching their TV was a concept I abandoned as too awful to believe. Yet I found a way to fight: I put ¼ of the *lad* into a film-noir television broadcast where they got sealed into drums and buried in about 1936... another ¼ chased a chocolate "Star

Bar" out of the living-room window... and the *ratnika* went into an empty lager can, with a glass on top that had a note in it facing down wards, saying "Beer Tomorrow"! It had indeed been a grand effort, but I didn't get rid of them all. The sensation of spores washing around in my body probably helped me get to sleep – and logically the enemy didn't want that. One morning I woke up and they were gone.

This book is an expansion of memories re-drafted from my first hand-written version of *Defender: Adventures in Schizophrenia*. It is precious to me, but memory itself is particularly precious to *feelie souls*. In this example a space-ship called "Cronenberg's Brick" started sucking up minds and I needed to *Cabal* him because he was attacking the memories of *feelies*. The problem of memory manipulation was solved later when the *feelies* themselves began painting pictures of their recollections. At this juncture my testament amounted to little more than a few pages of disconnected scribbles and a couple of times I entertained the possibility that if the *feelies* could not write and lost their memories everything that I had personally said and done – every battle, opinion, and revelation – would be wiped out as though they had never been. I couldn't face the erasure of the last five months, having to answer of all those Q & As, again. So I *caballed* the representative of Cronenberg until his space-craft accelerated off to the mysteries of somewhere else.

By that month most memories of my dog were also gone. I had believed she was a reincarnation of a Charlie from a passed 'policy' and she had gunned strange symbols at me like ankhs and stars, from her furry forehead, which I felt hit my brain physically. She certainly made a cute 'artillery piece'! My air-mattress got a puncture so I forced myself into town to buy another one. Into the mail went a parcel of personal items to Charlie, near the time of a miraculous event. A metal screw from a microphone was *teleported* from Radio One into Flat 12, and Charlie found a piece of Beaky

Bird food which had materialised from my flat to hers. It was interesting... but life in Thornfield Court was going into a skid. It was becoming a mess and I was eating bowls of beans and cold pork luncheon-meat from the tin.

Since Charlie worked for BBC Radio One there were a few friend-destroying vave-sims going on, as you might expect, about others who worked there... D.J Mark Goodier was an 'E' man, also, who made the occasional relaxing universe... D.J Andy Kershaw had no girlfriend, so I used a *long reach* to build up his confidence – and he went off happier...

D.J Jo Whiley was using erotic rapture (given to her by Barker when she had been young) to intercept my letters to Charlie – so I thought. When I had the courage to ask I telephoned the reception and learned it was a baseless allegation. In a leap of belief verging insanity I discovered some of their rooms and offices had been copied, identically in the *Helter Incendo* and that some of the D.J.s couldn't tell the difference. This may have been possible during the night, when the enemy set to work on people in their sleep, but somehow I believed it was also happening during the day! It's a good example of the awesome manipulative power of a *swit* enforced simulation, especially in my state of increasing weakness.

Some personal revelations put myself on a pedestal – a re-incarnation of Jesus with an internal history made up of six and a half entire genetic circles that could account for every life I have led for billions of years. After a last material plane adventure, stealing CDs from a record fair, the really bad *vave-sims* took off. I got away with a *Café Del Mar* compilation, maybe a *St.Etienne*, maybe another copy of a double set of ambient trance music, and about three CDs by *R.E.M* – that I sneaked past the dealers in the bag when I was slung out onto the street! That month I found my left eye was getting weaker. I was worried it was under rapture attack. A force of police officers (*aliens*) approached me from a rear vicinity and did experiments. The answer revealed itself. I had been wearing two right lenses at once: a weaker lens in the higher prescription left eye so it was sorted out.

Barker was stretching the distance of my 'broadcast' in a bid to rally forces against me. Apparently he wanted to destroy everything to save himself. Obviously I tried to stop this, but he threw blood and fire down the time-lines: made terrifying wars on the populated planets, annihilated *feelie* planes, and was creeping up on the last Time Asgaroth that could undo it. The Lords on that panel could cancel the horrors, so a desperate effort began to prevent the time-lines involving Barker's destruction being launched. He gate-crashed onto the seat at the 2.9, the last stop, and locked out any rescue package. All was lost. Looking back at a universe crinkling itself into a gigantic *incendo,* called a *'mat wah'* to become nothing, Barker was to stand there alone forever in blackness. A part of Stamp was put in the 'mat-wah' to over-dose him on blood. This was a tour-de-force vave-simulation – and may also have been a clue to the nature of the *Helter Incendo*. Peloquin and The Editor fought their war with integrity. Compared to the con-artists and liars that were supposed to be on their side, honour was everything to them. Emerging after I'd sometimes "had a hard day at the office", either, or both of them, used to bid me goodnight. They occasionally said that the day had been a good fight, if indeed it had been... and they even gave me the idea, once, that I might win. A woman used to shout, regularly: "It's a job!"

Britain's telepath forces were centralised in London. I saw occasional words or phrases in the night sky from that direction and occasionally on TV. I believed they were being fed nonsense from huge 'sub-thought cannons' attached to the side of the house, which were over thirteen feet high. On the roof was a kind of 'score-board' presenting the percentages of life, the odds of death, statistics about Earth survival, and other 'information' that I only ever saw by *looking up* underneath it from an angle. At the end of October such 'technology' was redundant. The 1997 battle of Halloween was about my home-spun white rapture against practitioners of the Black Arts. I assumed I would be fighting against witches of the United Kingdom, first, then I would lock swords with those in America the next night - but I got the dates back to front and inaccurate by many hours. As it turned out only one conflict mattered: that of the U.K.

Preparing my defence I plucked a white October rose from the garden, and mixed its fresh petals into granules of melting wax. I dropped the stubs of some old *Candles of Hope* into the mixture then tore open a tea bag, and sprinkled the dried leaves into the apparatus I stirred on the stove. Then I poured much of it into a mould shaped like Santa Claus. I placed the nine blue vortex paintings round the flat, with a bulwark affect facing outwards, and then rubbed raw magic wax in the corners of doorways and windows as further shielding. My rapture candle was the colour of ochre chocolate and it crackled with little sparks when it was lit. I did a lot of shifting about, and muttering. At near 11:38pm a dark bear shape swept past me.

Some called it a *Balrog*. A demon. It passed by my position just inside the living-room doorway. Although I saw it, before it disappeared out of the window, it could not have been a hallucination because there was a power outage when it brushed the TV and stereo plugs. At that exact instant a socket blew with a flash of smoke and the plug was carbonised. It makes you wonder how much of the rest of my story is also facts. Maybe I need extra medication. Don't ask me I only work here!!

By that November a few things were clearer to me. The perverse life-style I had led in the mid-nineties had been a retro-active character-assassination. I know that because the enemy later brought up some of the more sordid aspects of my history. I had felt strongly toward Barker then and wanted, for several years, to die with him in a nuclear flash. This indicated I had been driven almost to the opposing pole of what I was to stand for. On learning the truth of the beast I became his enemy. Barker had *wanted* me to hate him. In the title page of *Cabal* is the ink-press of two noble creatures, linked by the hands, twin-like. It is an attractive fiction. There was no equality in our actual capabilities. Wrong reflectively yet true conceptually: myself as white, truth, love and heterosexual for women – and Barker, as black, lies, hate, and homosexual for men.

The enemy told me that Sharlene Spiterie was imitating Charlie Jordan. I was under the impression that others on her side didn't like Sharlene much either. "Call me spit," she asked, but I couldn't see any beautiful woman in a disparaging light. Especially not someone I had muddled with Charlie. The four of us could perhaps be pictured in the easy metaphor of a Yin-Yang construction. Barker was the large black half, the area known as the *Daxial*, and I was the *Paxial*, the large reflected white side. Charlie represented the *Pixie*, the white spot trapped in the black, and Sharlene was the small black *Dixie* in the white. I wrote in my original diagram that Satan was the Deyaform and the god of the Earth was the Asgaroth. "Are you ready to let yourself drown? Are you holding your breath?" sang Sharlene on the album *White on Blonde*. "A secret screams so loud… You let me believe that you are someone else. So let me believe that I am someone else." That is what she sang.

The *Daxial* of Barker had a mortal fear for his soul and a lot of guilt. He would destroy me as utterly as possible if he couldn't have me. The women had been groomed for this situation for years. Israel was the place I had said I would die, thus a strong link, which caused an awakening within me when I heard the name *Jordan*. I also thought of the possibility that Charlie was 'bi' sexual. In the song *'Home'* by Depeche Mode they sang: "a cage or the heaviest cross ever made, the gauge of the deadliest trap ever laid." I hadn't known what Charlie actually looked like and when I masturbated about her that spring I had been manipulated into seeing Charlie's face in that of a photograph of Sharlene. Charlie was a lovely woman to me and a thorn trapped in Barker's side – the little white spot in the black – which could be seen as the girl-friend trapped in the *Helter Incendo*. Sharlene was the gay woman stuck in me, wanting Charlie for herself, sharing a mutual fear with Barker of their being stuck together 'after'. I rarely considered the complications of our *feelie* souls having differing genders to our bodies to explain our sexual orientations. I needed Charlie to contact me in *vicinity one,* in the Material Plane, but I was a 'joe' with a psychiatric record stretching back seven and a half years!

There had been other *Asgaroth / Deyaform* configurations drawn up over those months. The real trap might have been to believe it. Yet 'then' I believed that some had been constructed long ago. Barker had lied and shuffled people around for over two decades. He had engineered the telepath mythology that the celebrities needed. Because my apocalyptic belief had tallied with his for so long 'the end' might have seemed to be dreadfully unavoidable. The cyclic nature of it assisted acceptance and there had been much talk of swapping lives in the 'next policy triax'. They also said I was to be an integral cause. But how could I have caused anything? I had no power. I had enough problems trying to find my next dirty magazine! 'After' meant after an Armageddon. And no one wanted it. So since that July, when I had said: "I'm not going to cry for the Earth anymore," hope sprang from an unexpected place. I became an Earth *Defender*.

As I have written before the real conflict revolved around the creation and destruction of belief. 'Mind life' opinion and due respect was important. The belief that my *Reacher* was accurate, the belief I was capable of my own decisions, and the belief that those decisions were based on my own instincts – none were true. Vave-sims generated conviction in nonsense and a nightmare life-style through their evolution. But I kept going. The Quiddity structure of the Los Angeles vicinity 'Everville' was a lucid-dream destination. Telepaths could continue working on projects there in their sleep. I believed this Quiddity spirit, which had been used to create 'Everville', had been a legacy Barker had stolen from me using a 'spinal tap' that caused a terrible back-ache for twelve years. 'Everlie' (as it has also been called) was connected to my lounge via the 'Dream Corridor'. My ceiling had been dissolved into another place and surrounded by rapturers on top of the walls. They were dropping little scraps down onto me like radio-active shits, in a *'Wykera Pit'*. After my 'sublim' had washed away their insect *feelies,* it was packed up. I'm not chronologically sure about when, but it was dismantled.

In November when I was taking a bath I learned the Time-lord, Jon Pertwee, was dying from lack of sleep and poisoning. The enemy had inflicted him with coffee matter-collectors (*nussifyers*) so he had drank a crushing weight of caffeine to satiate them but just made himself sick and tired. I guided him into a shower and ejected the *nussifyers*. Soon after a cup of hot black tea, the traditional drink for a Time-lord, he went off happier to bed and he slept well. With multiple-vicinity techniques in 'time-turning' he became a powerful ally. I have believed worse: a *Helter Incendo* planet had once burned the Earth for sixteen years.

Uprising souls in an *Incendo* were pulled back down to die repeatedly in a reversal of heaven. It had been Hell itself. In that 'now' some cities were under huge sealed domes of *Dimension Two*, the muck containing the crumbled bones of old policies. Harlan Ellison wanted his people in the principal *Incendo* areas to wear uniforms like Nazis. There was a

195

movement of revolutionaries led by Mr. Sean Bean that fought with the musket riffles of the Sharpe series. My faith that Charlie and I would be together one day was twisted into something terrible. I never knew how to free her from this potential Hell until I came across a battle against it, which took me over seven hours to fight.

On November 15th 1997, I was sitting on the air-mattress in my bedroom and found myself engaged in a conflict against the entire *Incendo* vicinity. Something akin to a lawn mower (driven by someone I never knew) charged through the place tearing up the Dimension Two, which kicked up clumps of 'birds'. They might have been flying escape vehicles that attacked in formations, peeling off like in a dog-fight, and I destroyed them using home-spun hand raptures for finite targeting. They burst into rounded marbles of black anthracite that the enemy tried to collect. While rolling down corridors, themselves being torn up, I thrashed the anthracite with thought waves. Enjoyable and physical, like hand-cranking the barrels of an antique Gattling gun, I smashed the marbles revealing a drop of blood in each. The battle was a frenzy of crashing and smashing until about seven hours later (and having had only two and a half cigarettes) there was almost nothing left of it but hundreds of gallons of blood. The Enemy 'memory return' initiative failed because there wasn't enough *mass* left to work with. This was good, but this battle had been a 'singularity': It could not be repeated. After the victory, I got into my summertime bag and went to sleep. I drifted off with a sense of achievement and I got up late.

This was to be a different kind of day. A few *scu* wandered around the ruins of the *Incendo*. I told them to project love and cuddles at what remained. The Dimension Two softened and fell away like old porridge. I figured the *scu* were free to leave what was mostly just a platform above a huge gaping hole in the ground of *vicinity two*. My lingering sense of victory turned to my telepath girlfriend Charlie, who I called Charlotte. Troubling me was what Material Plane excuse could legitimise her contact with a besotted fan? I didn't think it was a serious problem. In a way that was typical of me I thought it would work itself out. The obvious method of communication, as I had suggested in a love letter, was to record her first greetings into a microphone.

On a connected *scu*-line that afternoon Charlie came to me on a real time 'live' link called an *inter-lace*. She had news and was buzzing like heavy electric cable. I went to the mirror in the bathroom so she could see me through my eyes. Her excitement was infectious. We kissed through the glass and she said she had done it, she had finally done it! She had recorded a tape for me! It was as amazing as stopping the Niagara Falls to take a bath. Yet... suddenly, I felt her absolute terror! She was shouting. The shock of it blew our happiness apart like a grenade. Her house was being broken into. She was screaming about men with knives. I became traumatised, suddenly feeling the cuts that her assailants were inflicting upon her. I stumbled to the vicinity-mesh of where she lay dying on my bedroom floor and part of her was with me, part of me with her.

I could feel the cuts to her face as heat in my own cheeks. And out of nowhere came the thought these scars might spoil my feelings for her, that it would be better if she died. The thought had been accompanied by an embarrassment that in her extremis wasn't sane. Later I tried to dismiss this as an attack *sub-thought*, but die she did. Her *feelie* suddenly bolted upwards like a rocket-star. She went the 'long way' around the planet passing a huge cage of bodies twisting and writhing in a Hell called *Mandar*, and then she found the heavenly stack, above and beyond that, of *feelie* Asgaroths. I lost contact. She was safe. And my own decision had been made: I would also die.

My left wrist was testament enough to the legacy of a blundered episode of self-harming and I wouldn't go off the 'Y' balcony because I had promised Charlie I wouldn't do that. Even if the oath was no longer binding I was terrified of falling. I was growing infirm from a lack of sustenance so I decided I would 'fade'. Stop eating and die in my sleep from malnutrition aided by a lack of will to live. I was tired of fighting and planned to be with the soul of my beloved Charlotte by Christmas. It felt like I had been on holiday for too long and wanted to go home. I 'went soft' by the gas fire a lot. Heaven is made of beautiful dreams, but if I experienced any normal dreams or 'visions' during those long sleeps I don't remember them.

CHAPTER EIGHTEEN – <u>DECEMBER: 1997</u>

One of the worst *vave-sims* of December involved a mortal threat to Charlie's *feelie*. Less a soldier then, more a lover in terror of her loss, I rose to her defence. Once again there was a deadly aerosphere withdrawal but this time our planet's *Deyaform* rotator disengaged simultaneously. I felt the pitch and yaw of the Earth while I was sitting in the lounge as it rolled along the Solar System in a state of gravitational collapse. Our air was being sucked up into another planet's siphon Gate and people started to die. Andrew, my neighbour downstairs, *scu'd* in to tell me that he was one scared telepath. It was good to have him on board.

Spaceships capable of destroying souls began skirting the Earth's atmosphere. They were rectangular blocks red-hot underneath like clothing irons. I could smell the burning of souls dashing against their undersides. They were becoming dust. Charlie's *feelie* bolted to me for protection. The craft had the worst name, quite the worst expression I had yet heard: they were *Air Incendiary Vehicles*. I had a brick-down area inside my right arm that was like a bed of cotton wool. Charlie hid in it. I was terrified. It felt like I was sitting on a beach ball floating out to the sea. The Gates sucked and the machines blotted up rising souls. Believing the inconceivable threat in that upward tugging, I held my right arm tightly against my ribs to prevent the total loss of my loved one.

There was an unclear connection between Harlan Ellison and *Air Incendiary Vehicles*. I posted a diagram of a cross-section of one of the machines against the living-room wall with the ghost of a *sub* that someone had *allowed me* to. Before I could decide that Andrew and I might be some of the last people left alive, I inspired some souls into an act of bravery that I didn't grasp myself: to charge and ram the undersides of the attack ships. Perhaps it was an answer controversial enough for the enemy to talk about afterwards for a long time. The *Incendiary vehicles* broke up as souls rammed them hard and fast and blew them to pieces.

Of course the entire fight had been a typically unbalanced *vave-sim*, yet I discovered it had been a re-enactment of a past Policy during which Ellison himself had invented the machines. It had been an annihilation that only a monster could conceive but it had been wonderful that it had never actually happened, then. I went to bed when all was clear; Andrew *scu'd* back to himself and Charlie went back to hers. I was asleep when the sun, against the odds (if you consider what had taken place the night before) did actually rise in the morning.

The moment a *vave-simulation* becomes a reality crisis is when incontrovertible evidence of it exists physically in *vicinity one*. In the first half of December I found a sore spot growing on the left side of my tongue. Hurting as it grew, my attention was drawn to it and to 'subtle bodies' somehow condemned to a *nullility escent tank* that were escaping through a tiny hole – perhaps 'meshed' with that hole in my sore ulcer – so small worms emerged into my mouth, later known as "tongue wah". I spat one on to my lounge coffee table and watched it. It was one centimetre long, two millimetres wide, and clear-bodied except for markings that may have been vertebral. They had an astonishing ability of sliding along for about seven inches before sinking into the wood and vanishing. I heard a famous model was in hospital with the same problem. Her *scu* was repeatedly carrying them back to my tongue and I didn't think the inevitable quarantine was going to hold.

I decontaminated the worm gate with the help of four aliens on a *brick-down* in the knuckles of my right hand. They were called *Barks*, males that reproduce amoebically: splitting off a baby in the same way as their lesbian enemies, the *Alphas*. Bark religion involved *rapture* and they didn't seem to want to stand back while the Earth people died and went up crazy with no tongues. They taught me to use an image made solid: that of a small flat spike on my index finger that I pushed into the ulcer, with applications of toothpaste. The gate closed, the worms stopped coming. Two days later a piece of convex flesh fell out of my tongue where the ulcer had been. It was a solid tissue firing mechanism and its absence left a gap that had never felt so good!

After Beaky had flown away my mother replaced him with the most vicious looking cockatiel I had ever seen. I had seen quite a few in the shops and this one looked like death warmed up. He had beady little eyes and a great gnarled beak that was as sharp as an arrow tip and as strong as the bow that fired it. I called him 'War Bird' but he drew blood at the first opportunity and disappeared under circumstances that were never clear. I found a note in my hand from the Colchester Police regarding a small dog that had been found, most likely Lotti, but in my state of exhaustion I couldn't make the connection in my mind. I couldn't tie it together, could hardly even remember her. The air-mattress got a puncture so I set up four bean bags in a row in the bedroom. I slept there in my duvet, or in the lounge. I woke up to a 'hunger-striker's breakfast' of a cigarette and a cup of tea every morning – assuming that it actually was 'morning' when I got up – and I had been known to say about smoking, ruefully: "These things'll kill you!"

I re-patched the Devine force of the 'silver shield' Kaos linkage through an antique silver brooch that was itself shaped like a shield. I pinned it to a stolen woolly hat. I hadn't eaten a Sunday dinner at my parents for months and had barely cooked five of my own meals since October. My *reacher* had been copied for use as a weapon on alien spaceships. The brooch started to hurt my frontal cerebral hemisphere so I took it off. A few Alphas visited and I found myself talking some of the ladies' language. Their ringed planet was *Alpha Centauri,* 5.2 light years away, "two days down the alley at light-speed", according to telepaths at Goonhilly Tracking Station. It had a pink sky, a perfumed atmosphere and orbited a Red Dwarf Star, hidden behind our sun, called Betelguise. I enjoyed talking their language but most of the time I couldn't have cared less if my *reacher* had been made into a toaster.

That December the nights and days had both been dark: a fantasy of death, of visits from Charlie and cuddling in the murk, losing myself. She told of *feelies* 'bean venting' to make things more 'realistic', and told of adventures skimming *vicinity zero* (she'd once been rescued from outer space!) and about *scunes*. These could visit you in your last days, were recorders that could enable you to carry things with you up to Heaven – a device I believed Charlie had invented herself! I soon gave up any record of shoes or clothes. I decided that all I really wanted up there was my soft pillow Fred.

The enemy used to ask: "where do you go when you sleep?" and it worried me. Because if I died as I wanted, during slumber, the enemy could trap my soul and the forces of goodness might not know it had even happened. An answer had to be found. Apparently the volume of my broadcast telepathy, such as birds singing in the mornings, was louder to them than when I was awake, which started me thinking about music. I had avoided the band R.E.M for years; the spikes on the album cover of *Automatic for the People* had been like a gigantic STOP sign. Yet that winter I had three CDs by the band: *The Best of R.E.M*, *Reckoning*, and *Out Of Time*. I believed their songs incorporated a hidden rhythm that encouraged sleep, a subliminal 'click track' matching human REM pattern waves – hence the name R.E.M. I decided I would 'sleep-down' playing their songs. When the music stopped I would be dead.

One night I had a dream of an ancient history that may have been the source of The Garden Of Eden legend. An exciting recognition awoke me with lingering visions of eons long past. I remembered when our family had lived on a spacecraft, when Charlotte and I had been brother and sister telepath aliens wanting to kiss each other but we had little gaping mouths and no tongues. I suppose we must have looked a bit like 'Teletubbies". Our parents may have been Sharlene and Barker and we had lived in a classic shaped flying saucer named *The Gut*. Pronounced 'goot' it had tubular corridors lit by the brightness of glowing blocks of crystal and a Quiddity pool on board that we called 'pluria'.

Charlie's *feelie* arrived to discuss these fascinating recollections. I leant over the edge of the air-mattress to sketch the control room and write details. We recognised ancient expressions like, "The cubulars shin-ath", and "A wim in the pluria", and food parcels called "Silver-packs." The story goes that taking a dip in the Quiddity, on our last day on *The Gut,* Charlie and I had shared a dream of different bodies. We became aware of one another's nudity and it may have taken place in a lovely garden, and there may have been an apple involved that in modern myth represents *The Art.* Our parents discovered our sexual congress. When they saw a red mist rising from the Quiddity pool Charlie and I were kicked off *The Gut* into outer space and died. This wasn't so much a *vave-simulation* as the fabrication of memory applied live on a full *scu*-lock.

I have written that many vave-sims were about the macro-cosm being '*bricked down*' into the micro-cosm and I came across quite a believable example of this in mid-December when Charlotte told me about a huge structure: a universe comprised of sixty-four huge rectangular blocks with sixty-four galaxies on the front of each. Each block was three hundred light years from either side to the middle, the galactic plates had Deyaform timing and Asgaroth holding – cells. The whole thing was in a sphere coated in protective silver that had come from my 'K' link, which had become called the Shield Dome. Charlie was living in the centre of one of these blocks and she called it her 'space set'. The fear of a larger enemy existing outside the Shield Dome was destined to become a vave-sim later, in 1998.

One afternoon I sealed up the flat and placed a lit candle on a shelf, in a far corner of the living-room while the heater was gushing unlit propane. I must have assumed that my neighbours were out working at the time because I got tucked up in soft stuff to 'sleep down' in a room that was effectively a bomb. But I couldn't sleep so I opened the doors and some windows; and, after ensuring it was free of gas, I lit a cigarette and drank some tea. Potentially worse self-harming than what I had done to my hand on 2nd April, it was the closest I had been to death since the suicide attempts of rope, wrist, and roof, in 1990 and 1991. I heard Charlie's show on the radio. It should have changed the entire situation but I thought the broadcast had been pre-recorded. No one directly told me that Charlie was alive.

I still wanted to be dead by Christmas but if precautions such as R.E.M music-sleep were not taken the enemy might pluck me like ripe fruit. Rapture me into any number of terrible fates; a tiny blind 'reacher-worm' searching for my loved one – a nothing in the blackness of nullility – or staring at a visual horror while suffocating in a box called an 'air-less photograph'. I washed ritually at night and wore white shirts to bed like shrouds. I prayed to wake up in Heaven but it was happening so slowly. In telepathic contact with a 'bad boy' from the BBC soap *Eastenders*, who was boss of a crime syndicate in London, I asked him to send two of his men down to Colchester to shoot me. When I heard they had arrived I walked downstairs, wearing my dressing gown and clasping a wooden cross. I walked out onto the pavement ready to get it done. There were a couple of people further down the road, but no guns. I went back upstairs to my cloistered death-throws in the filthy mess of scratched CDs and rubbish littering the flat for a smoke and a cupper.

One night I unintentionally moved us out of the normal 1.2 Time-line (of sixty seconds per minute / sixty minutes per hour) so the planet became dimensionally out of synch. Lost in time. It was like trying to leave the grid reference of a crashing aeroplane: "This is an S.O.S from planet Earth... our time position is now on the Starion Asgaroth at 2.9... Can you hear me? Shifting now towards the 3.2... S.O.S! Can anyone hear me? Hello?!" Sitting at the coffee table I felt like a hack D.J during an Ice Age, riding the Earth like a bucking bronco trying to lock us back onto normal time. About an hour later help did arrive. A crowd emerged from a *brick-down* door in my mind called an *Inter-Gate* led by Lord Jon Pertwee. They were shouting and waving signs and the Time Lord quickly plugged us back into *vicinity one*. I didn't realise my digital watch was displaying a date that was actually five days ahead of everyone else!

"Never make an oath" is generally good advice – which I didn't follow. *'Pushed'* easier in my weakened state I said if I ever smoked again I would pull off the ring that represented my love for Charlie and burn it. I lit a candle and set it atop the coffee table. Within half an hour my chest area was so full of nicotine, *nussifyer*, 'matter-collectors' that the dreadful urge for a cigarette was physically painful. I lit up and put the ring into the candle flame but a higher force stopped me because the withdrawal had been engineered. The oath was declared void. I reclaimed the ring, which was silver with about eleven Yin-Yang sets embossed around it, and it slipped it back on my finger.

I decided to ask some army telepaths to assist my death. Colchester is a garrison town. They offered to shoot gas canisters through the living-room front window but that would have been so loud it would have made a 'sleep-down' impossible. The soldiers then said they could pipe it through the fire-vents, and I agreed. I was awake and worried about the neighbours when they put the nerve gas through, but I was told it was a short-range weapon. I was ready for the crossing like a wrecking ball about to demolish a dividing wall, and I knelt waiting for the smell that would crumple me into a nerveless heap and kill me after eleven months of telepathy. It failed. When another second poison was tried I fancied I could actually smell it. It had a scent like bleach, but that failed also. Would I accept cyanide…? An insane pain but for barely eight seconds…? I told them: "yes!" and then I prepared for an agony that never came. I had survived again, and had the sense to open the doors and windows before I calmed down with tea and cigarette.

One night I lit some little candles around the living room and Charlie's *feelie* came down for an expression of love perhaps as physical as is possible for a couple on a *two-in-one*. We had a short time of great happiness in what became called *'The Room of the Five Candles'*. We were privately connected by a rapture each called Love Talkie Pearls, effervescent spheres connecting and reflecting one another's sensate physicality. In the musk and flickering light I became content and aware of romance while cuddling, and I was shown an image of the outside of the room like a drifting box. Later it was claimed to have been visualised in a *nullility* tank seen through a blue filter, but what I saw then was the scintillating wake of our love floating behind our room like bubbles.

I hadn't eaten a nourishing meal for over sixty days. I continued to weaken. My 'reality tunnel' was a long darkness feeble as the summer dreams of a hibernating squirrel. I have never woken up on Christmas morning with a girl-friend before but it seemed likely that I would that year. I would share this special time with Charlie in her Heavenly 'space set' that was decorated with a Christmas tree adorned with a complete archive of memory cards from my previous lives. One early afternoon I came across a stainless steel bowl of fresh water, with a lettuce leaf draped over it. I thought of a large cup of Quiddity and a soft duvet and it was funny. I fell on the floor perhaps still smiling with sudden motor-failure. I playfully imagined myself being stuck on the ceiling looking 'down' and it could be said that I faked dying – but the faint, which had dropped me to the floor in the first place, had been quite real.

In a hot relaxing bath with the room lit by a few flickering flames, I relaxed, maybe muttering to myself. I did that often. Since July had been using my voice box instead of a 'Talk-box'. My eyes drifted… and a candle flame became a bubble through which I saw aliens bidding me goodbye: A hallucination of Alpha perfume ladies, Cyclops, Barks and maybe some *feelies*. I had another faint and my temple hit the bath enamel. I saw an exit gate in the bottom right corner of my vision, a new gate: if it had been blue rather than red, if the enemy had been reassuring, (in spite of my legendary instinct for survival that I developed later) things may have been different. But anyone can say "What if?" anytime, about anything, and gain nothing. Once again the initial faint had seemed real. I was sinking, doubtfully, but I felt a bolt like electricity through my chest and 'came to'. I saw a woman turning away, an apparition with curly hair carrying heart-defibrillators, one in each hand, and I leapt out of the bath. Even if I had been nowhere near dying I still saw this woman – and she still gave me treatment for what most medical staff would call a 'Code Blue' cardiac arrest – so again I was a survivor. I had my hunger-striker's breakfast, of course, but life was not what I wanted.

My capability for manipulating telepathy and maybe a few other faculties were sucked out during an attack by five Air-Gates: four in the walls and a huge one in the ceiling. I saw them tear a glittering torrent of gold dust out of the top of my head while I was 'watching myself from the side'. One of the questions the enemy may have asked one another is…Would they actively *assist* in my death that December? Since I was seeking it, their physical action may have been seen as more of a helping hand than 'an attack'. I don't know I did not have the Big Picture. It may have prevented their serious intervention but if *push-sub-thoughts* could fill my room with flammable gas maybe other physical intrusions were unnecessary? I didn't think enough about what could go wrong after I died, until my back was against the wall. I told attending telepaths I had seen the *Universe Generator* filled with 64,000 airless-photographs. The possibility that my death might harm others, globally, could have been used as a blackmail excuse to live. Maybe I did that later on, and needed to reconcile a flash of *push-sub* embarrassment, but when I focussed on living it was usually about the long future. Good aspects of survival: the end of firearms; the invention of light-speed engines.

It had been the year when Barker had let rip his war-machine while he was writing 'Galilee'. Business went as usual for him, while I was rapidly sinking into oblivion. My metabolism must have been exceptionally slow. I wasn't getting thin but I seemed to be falling into unconsciousness instead of sleep. One night I woke up at 9:30pm, got off the bean-bags, walked like a zombie into the kitchen to drink water; then went back to sleep. I 'came to' at 9:30pm the next night – again – for more water from the kitchen tap then returned into that dreamless disintegration. Finally I found myself wandering into the kitchen into a blazing sun, dawn shining bright into my face, at about 6:45am. It was a new day. I praised the Lords above for getting me through the darkness and I had my usual 'breakfast', which hadn't tasted so good for ages!

Of course I forgot Christmas cards but in more lucid moments I had been making notes about the on-going battle that I faxed to Radio One. The following night I sent the whole package to every telepath machine receiving on the planet, in what they were calling a 'fax-bus'. The jump-point for this was through Colchester's local radio station S.G.R. I had a hic-cup with it when I thought I had sent the data through the machine without the telephone cable plugged into the wall, but it wasn't a miracle. For certain it was received by SGR.

Another fascination was when I found some presents wrapped up and waiting for Christmas day. Either of my parents could have dropped them off, to flat 12, if I had let them know I wouldn't be with them. Survival with these presents might make the short future with Charlie a little more special! On my own private Christmas 'Eve (days early due to my faulty watch) I had a feast. I walked down to the shop with my cheque-book and purchased pork pies, cheeses, sweet tarts, fruit mince pies, milk, tomatoes, cakes, steak and kidney pies, chocolate, chicken and mushroom pies, sweet slices, soft drinks and crisps. A similar list – or maybe more! If you suspect any exaggeration I can tell you for a fact that I wrote a cheque that evening for over sixty pounds! I laid out the spread and sensed a joy from within, maybe from others 'without'. My happiness was contagious to interior *scu*, pleasing, and sometimes it had also been revelatory although never for long. Unfortunately, the remainder of that night was when my wedding came undone.

I wore sacrificial white on the beanbags and prayed to awaken with Charlie's *feelie* soul in her latest place, a small Quiddity home. She told me to hurry up so we could be married on Christmas morning – and I was looking forward to it with excitement. I hoped I had retained a weakness sufficient enough to be fatal. I asked for my wrists to be 'mack'ed (with pulse-interrupters) but I had eaten a lot and couldn't even get to sleep. So I lay back and felt the rear of my brain being squeezed hard with an inter-dimensional hand. If I remember rightly it had been the hand of David Cronenberg, a painful crushing sensation for which he had even apologised. In her house Charlie found a white wedding dress upstairs, waited for me for a while, then went up to try it on. *Feelies* that looked like 'Teletubbies' were coming into the garden. She didn't know what to do about them and they were upsetting her.

I suspected they were sexually curious; they started climbing up the walls. Charlie was getting so unhappy, the emotionally sensitive Quiddity structure of the house started to decay. The *feelies* were peering into the windows and climbing over the flimsy roof, while the walls were dripping with slime. In a typically horrible *vave-sim* our house was demolished through highly charged emotions; crumpled up, fell to the ground in a heap of dust and slimy shrapnel. I rose from the beanbags. I watched TV and drank tea to sober up from the experience and knew that because of my Christmas feast a 'sleep-down' was impossible. The entire After-Life thing was in disarray.

Having accepted being alive I could at least look forward to opening my presents the next day with Charlie on a *two-in-one*. Fast adaptability is one of my strong suits, the 'bounce'. On the carpet between the heater and the coffee table I shovelled the empty food, cigarette packets, crap, ashtray spills, rubbish, scratched CDs and cracked cases under the table with my right foot to clear a space for a nest. I slept.

Christmas is one of my favourite holiday seasons. It's like a huge family birthday yet so many previous celebrations have passed me by with little memory of the magic we had shared. The recollections went into that dark place of deceased history like the ashes of a burnt photo album. 25th December to me, was about the 19th to everyone else and the wrapping paper made happy crackling noises as I tore it off the presents. I got some clothing and a beautiful wooden box of oil-colour tubes, with brushes. A 'disappointment' *sub-thought cannon* (standard Christmas issue) dwelt on the fact that I don't like using hog's hairbrushes, but it didn't dent the best gift of all. I was given a glittering crystal tortoise, which I placed on a red cushion by the east-facing window in my bedroom. Other surprises were not so good: the Police arrived two days later.

They had come to ask questions about the Fax I had sent to S.G.R and they saw the wreckage. The place looked like a landfill site and it didn't smell good either. They left quickly but I had probably been earmarked for psychiatric assessment. My family doctor came in to take a look at what was left of my home and myself. I explained the mess had been caused during a party and shouted at him to "fuck off!" a few times. He went. But there was another party coming, a get-together with an enemy almost forgotten. The antagonist was the car thief I had lived with in Bristol in 1988, Paul Nicolau. The Greek Cypriot had adopted me as a kind of son to him and then terrorized me. I didn't know if I should have continued to cast him as an enemy, since I hadn't seen him for nine years, but I heard he was on the run and coming fast in my direction.

I recalled my fear. Looking into his eyes I had seen something there so black and so very deep I sometimes believed he was a soulless computer hiding a 'heads-up display' of complex grids. Usually there had been a part of me too terrified to define him – or think much of anything, like a fox frozen by car headlamps. The explanation I was given was that he was a lifeless 'X Card', a rapture card marked with a letter 'X' to accelerate his time-turning abilities instead of a soul. Paradoxically, after I may have ordered his death, there was a strong part of him still coming after me. He used a thirty-one piece 'pick set' that magnified the speed and affect of his rapture-board but it was me he wanted. He posed no threat to the *Shield Dome*. Like the worst power since the Gates he settled on inter-dimensional alchemy and altered my brain into black anthracite. I was told it was this and, in an inter-dimensional way, perhaps that is also what it felt like. And it was a trap.

Visiting *feelie* souls and *scu* were locking themselves into a disaster area. I shouted: "stay away!" but they were sucked into bricked-down pebbles and locked into the attack head where they suffocated. I went a bit crazy when I believed Charlie's *feelie* had also become trapped. Using 'K' linked imagination (not my 3D reading-drive, that was gone) I made a hammer that could connect with the same vicinity as the attack-head. I smacked the rock with it but just came up with fragments. I won the battle eventually. According to my original hand-written version of *Defender* I may have done it by putting myself closer to the fire and melting the anthracite like a ball of wax. In the peace treaty Paul agreed to take a job as a time policeman, beneath the Lords. Since he still had raptures in his arsenal it was a good arrangement. After a life of crime he might have thought it ironic to have wound up 'afterwards' as a Police Officer!

After Christmas there was a *vave-sim* about Simon Le Bon, about the legacy of his history applied to the present. In Roman times he had been a legionnaire named Simon Le Spartaclay, and he had treated Charlie so badly it defied belief. Of course the whole thing should have defied belief because I had been the voice from Simon's future. I told him while he was performing during a music show that his yacht 'Drum' was going to capsize in Cornwall, and he would get stuck underneath it. I warned him years *after* the event using telepathy during a song recorded on TV *before* the event, like a time-trick. I was jealous of him. Simon was living with Charlie at the top of a time spiral that was doomed because it wasn't circular.

The *feelies* there could see a gold ring in the sky, a cyanide prison circle that I was trapped in. In this scenario it killed me continuously for so many years the *feelies* forgot there was anyone in it. Yet the *vave-sim* was in defiance of suicide. There was so little I could do about it and after I somehow attracted the *feelies* attention to the ring, the *sim* was cancelled. In another I met two deities called "Quiddity Keepers", who, in order not to upset the spirit, spoke precisely and gently. The way they spoke seemed funny to me and soon they faded away too.

Then came the real 25th December, Christmas Day for everyone! I rode my motorcycle *'Erminscoot'* to West Mersea but I couldn't join my family initially because I hallucinated Mum with a tube emerging from a hole in her chest that went a very long way back in time. It was a funnel from a history of absent heart-boxes waving about ready to suck up as much inter-vicinity bits and pieces as it could get. I tied a knot in it. At the exact moment I walked into Dad's lounge my ears met with the same music that I had used to initiate new people into <u>The Harmonix</u> over eleven months before. *"Papua New Guinee"*, on the album 'Accelerator' by *Future Sound of London*. When I recognized it that day I felt a 'music rush' so powerful I believed it had vented all the evil out of the *Shield Dome*.

My mind was somewhere else then. I was incapable of properly sharing the celebration.
I had bought some presents for them but the answer to the exact 'when' and the 'how', is without much detail. My memories of the rest of that day are also gone. I rode back to Thornfield Court later that night. I remember another dark time when I might have witnessed the departure of my soul: the word L O V E written in glowing blue letters in the blackness. One by one they disappeared. The transition was

a part of the essence of the time, like being unable to swim and watching a diamond ring sinking into a lake. When the last two letters had faded that might have been the instant my soul had flown off to see Charlie.

They merged together on the top most Asgaroth of the *Feelie* Plains, that in their love they had rolled over and over and over as one, creating a ton of new Quiddity. And that is how it works, so I believed: souls living in beautiful dreams make new Quiddity, in their love for each other, for other lovers to have other beautiful dreams. I had a Chinese relaxation ball with six Yin-Yang sets on a background of glittering blue paint that contained a little bell. One day Quiddity may fill a gigantic sphere of six rotating universal plates, driven by music, containing only souls. With a beautiful optimism I called it the '*Feelie Ball of Wonder*'.

CHAPTER NINETEEN – <u>JANUARY: 1998</u>: *Hospital Five.*

I believed the days missing from the calendar had been because of Lord Jon Pertwee's *grand massive time-turns* that had affected the whole planet beyond the knowledge of its individuals. After I corrected my watch to the same date as everyone else's I rediscovered a thing forgotten. On New Year's Day I walked into my bedroom and found a shiny key beside a crystal tortoise sparkling in the late morning sun. It was a symbol of survival, glittering on a red cushion in the light shining through the east window, an allegory of moving to new pastures with your 'house upon your back'. I was with Charlie's *feelie* when I found it and I laughed so much I got the sub-thought I nearly died! When my chuckling was done I replaced the tortoise and the key wanting to do it again properly 'next time'. I saw a vision of two gold circles (perhaps signifying D.N.A circles and/or wedding rings) melt into a figure eight and then into one. It may have been an essence of marriage slipping away. Within days there was another miracle of survival but regarding the tortoise there was never to be a 'next time'.

I pumped over thirty minutes of cold propane into the living room through the hissing vent but I wasn't going to sleep during this one. I was going to be wide-awake and staring into the flames when the fire connected. In a room full of gas I knelt down with a box of matches, took one, and said: "Take my soul to God," and struck it. It lit, and I looked at the little flame for a moment before tossing it into the corner. It went out and there was no explosion. Before fetching my favourite calming formula I had to admit that I had been dauntless in this example. But when the enemy said it would have taken several minutes for me to die like that some of you might think it to have been conceptually stupid as well as 'brave'. Three days later it was a moot point because the Community Mental Health Team came up the stairs. I either pretended I wasn't in or swore at them, but part of me knew they would be back.

On the night of 4th January the Time Lords engineered the surprise release of ninety-nine 'past policy' Richards. I saw red visions from about 11pm, when the old souls were sprung from loops of their happiest moments. Yet they were far from happy. Almost all to a man seemed insane. I was trying to get to sleep and witnessed some dreadful memories. A dead baby called "Fred" – son of an ancient Richard – called Adrian Starliter who had pursued our enemy in the Material Plane with firearms, and other bloody oddities. When I finally slept

I experienced one soul's memory of a beautiful accidental meeting with his Charlie, when they had experienced that surge of happy recognition at first sight and moved with the onset of love. Through the dream I relived it. The memory had felt 'dusty' but I had believed the experience was mine. I awoke bereft.

The next day I studied the situation. I was looking for safe carriage to join my soul. "Blood death – that's our way!" said some old Richards, but I would not use a knife. I was looking for a way that was fast, certain, and simple. I knew it would have to be the "Y". I walked onto the upper landing while the enemy were working themselves into a frenzy of pros and cons on either side of the railing, and took a look at it – facing outwards, headfirst, twenty-seven feet to a cement floor: it would be mortally affective. My enemies were in confusions of dimension and thought called 'atom-smashes', spinning out of control, and oblivious of the opportunity to capture me so I got into position. By the time I was hanging upside down by my knees the posture was as inescapable as though I had already fallen. My heart was beating like the drums heralding a man to his gallows, and then some ancient Richards encouraged me to gradually loosen my knees. Dreadfully I began to slip... then fell. I flung out my right arm, smacked it on the edge of the steps, turned 170 degrees in mid-air, and landed on my left foot. I had gone headfirst off the "Y" balcony - and survived!

Nursing my injury I went upstairs to brew tea. I seemed to have sustained a broken arm but that fall should also have been 'it'. Bearing in mind I had nearly burned I was thinking that I was alive for a reason. I lit my cigarette and sipped my drink when the enemy told me nicotine and caffeine is poison in an open marrow wound, that it could be fatal. I believed them. I had to get help, physical help, and quickly. I rode a cab down to the A&E at the General and somehow forgot that my soul was already safe. On the ward, I started shouting with the desperation of approaching death and three possible dooms for an afterlife: an air-less crystal tortoise hanging in the black sky over Simon Le Spartaclay's limited 'heaven': nullifying to black nothing: or a blind 'reacher-worm' suffocating while trying to find where Charlie's screams were coming from while her legs were sawn off. I had taken similar damnations into consideration before but this time I was a dead man walking, already. So I went to the nurse's station and started shouting for help.

They said people were coming to see me. "Will they love me?" I asked, and they said they didn't know. A few minutes later two psychiatric nurses from The Lakes came in. They asked stupid questions, stupid because I wasn't suffering a mental illness: I had a broken-arm that was potentially lethal. Desperately needing physical help I swore at them until they went. Musing these unimaginable futures I was suddenly surrounded by uniformed policemen. Four officers took me outside, into the cold January night, and stood between my broken arm and treatment. They blocked the entrance to A&E, and I yelled something along the lines of: "Well kill me then for all the difference it'll make!" But even with no diagnosis of my arm, which they could not possibly have known, they didn't move. They were implacable as rock. Four standing stones erected to the misunderstanding of those who aren't deemed to be what society considers 'normal'. So I turned my back on them, and I started walking. I was looking for a couple of cigarettes and some strong tea that would be the easiest suicide in history.

I left a couple of butts and an empty pot cooling on a pub counter in North Station Road. I walked towards the town centre with a smile on my face; I didn't reckon I would see Thornfield Court again. I was expecting to just 'drop out' of life, literally, and suddenly, but I was still alive by the time I was waiting for a cab at a service just down St. John's Street from Vagabonds. My tactile drive that I rarely used was highjacked. I felt a wet ache, and a bad smell, and imagined a severe break through the skin. I knew this vision was an invention but I was still a little spooked. I didn't want to look at it and back at the flat I carefully peeled off my undershirt as gingerly as though unwrapping a dreadful gift from the forces of evil, true in some ways. In the dim light of the living room the skin was intact. I couldn't even see a bruise. I could move my fingers. The Time Lords said they would mend any small fractures while I slept, and sleep I did, but it had been a very 'hard day at the office'.

The night before I was led away a pellet was fired into my brain an inter-dimensional pellet that started growing. I could feel new skull plates forming that had the texture of cheese graters and I thought I was becoming a cyborg. I was to believe whatever they wanted me to for over sixteen more months. On the afternoon of 7th January the CMHT finally had me. Police officers backing up, social workers came through my front door with a battering ram. I heard the noises, sudden and loud. I felt like a trapped rat but I was lucid enough to secure my wallet and keys before they clamped on the handcuffs. The steel bracelets had hard edges and I was worried they might damage my tender wrist. I left the burst air mattress and the crippled CDs, the odour of dirty clothes and rubbish, behind, but not the war. Schizophrenia knows no bounds geographically. It is always evolving, and I was carrying it with me to The Lakes.

On arrival I was detained under Section Two of The Mental Health Act: four weeks involuntary treatment. It was the least

I could have expected. I would ensure I never ran out of tobacco products, disposed of medication, and interacted socially with the other patients. All part of a hospital 'set'. But I found that I had more on my plate than the boredom of such as wanting the kettle to boil faster. Within days I discovered the dread truth of the year, the placement in 1998 of attack 'spore'. Perhaps like 'nanobots' these spores are electrical devices so miniscule they can be transferred inter-dimensionally via a *fundament*. They came in differing sizes, are virtually invisible and split amoebically at different speeds. For example, "miniature two spore" are about the size of sperm cells yet collectively they feel large and dangerous to the robustness of the skull while dividing. The technology is both ancient and advanced. It is the result of runaway robotics so developed they had been deployed in wars against the living.

I was given a room beside the Nurse's Station. During one of my first nights I had an awful vision because of the weird crawling sensation of spore. Fuelled by ignorance I thought they were going to eat my entire head. A dreadful fate – particularly since I had been fighting the enemy that wielded them for ten and a half months – yet the next day I woke up. My parents brought along toiletries and clothes, and my pillow "Fred". The spore sometimes passed right through the 'cyborg head' and I guessed the new plates were for venting porously: giving me a chance? There was a metal hexagon at the base of the head and I didn't know if it was to vent or 'teleport'. Spore bombs, as Ellison called them, were arranged under the duress of miniature sci-fi creatures that looked like the enemy of Doctor Who, like tiny Cyber-Men, which were called 'spore-controllers'. I had little peace. I often thought at night that my head was going to explode in a cataclysm of injustice. In what became known as the *'Two Spore Incident'* my pillowcase contributed to saving me.

I've had a 'Fred Basset' pillow on my bed, with other pillowcases on and off, for over twenty years. Based on an early memory I have of not liking its texture when it was new to me as a child the truth maybe closer to being over twenty-five years. But it softened. Before losing my sense of smell I had enjoyed Fred's sleepy scent of hair and feathers and I also had a strong attachment to a thin grey pullover manufactured by Ben Sherman. The price tag had been lowered by five pounds, when I bought it, because the logo was back-to-front. I had an idea that an inverted logo might actually be worth quite a lot more than I paid for it, but I kept it because it was so comfortable against my skin that I called it my 'Softy Jumper'. About three years ago my mother found another 'Fred' pillowcase, in a charity shop, so I might carry his n' her 'Freds' from bed to bed in the future!

The *'Two Spore Incident'* began as most other nights did. My head was brimming with the dry metallic creeping of a large version two-spore occupation. The difference, in this example, was that the spore-controllers wanted to learn about people. Two exits were positioned on either side of the image: a gate to nullify Barker and a gate to nullify me. The controllers became judge, jury, and executioner. They ordered me to have an orgasm within ten minutes or die. I managed it and I thought that they would like the endorphins. I can't recall what else they asked about life and love, but they had a curiosity about Fred so I told them cuddly stuff also. They must have liked it because they agreed to leave porously. The horror was over. Dread left me like a long, slow sigh of relief – but in a twisted twist of fate I learned that the Large Two's were physically *too big* to porous vent.

Maybe it had all been a con from the start. Maybe it had been a torture dressed in poisonous frills – but whatever the reasoning behind it I was going to die anyway. I actually believed it had come about by accident. The controllers may have been apologetic in their way… and they would arrange a 'slow crack' while I slept. I drifted into the darkness of early morning. Felt stuff like foam on front top left of my head. Perhaps that had been a fracture, but the human skull is full of minute holes that can absorb an impact and it is as hard as rock. I lay there, not thinking much, drifting towards the new day. The sky brightened.

When the dawn sun shone red gold and beautiful through the window I went to the toilet. I found a small wet red stain on the material of 'Fred' but I noticed that there was no pressure inside my head like the night before. I walked into the linen washroom, for water to wash Fred and maybe to drink, and found Softy Jumper! I pulled it on and it felt good: a synchronous symbol, so I thought, of the Lord's help. I washed Fred. A remaining spore controller said the Type Two spore would never again kill a human being. For a while I was free. This had been a victory.

There are many factors involved when considering a universal size Yin-Yang configuration. If our Earth is represented by the small whiteness in the black half, you must also accept the existence of a black planet reflected in the Deyaform's mirror. I learned that it is called Antimax, an inversion of our planet. A small place in white space, as dry and polluted as our Earth is wet and green, because it has outlived us repeatedly in a dreadful tournament. When the universes' rotating mirror disengaged at the close of competition, Antimax's white space occupied the entire Asgaroth containment to our terrible cost. So its technology became hyper advanced, outlived our beautiful rich planet so many times it became a lifeless place occupied by robots, spore dust, and technology gone mad. And it was after *me*.

I was shot with pellets of a particular horror, of contagious spore that can be carried in the air called sub-drives, shooting them straight through the universal Deyaform into my head – with a gun the size of a house. I actually ran around the ward believing the pellets could be stopped if I hid behind walls and fire extinguishers! "Put your head in the toilet and let your head detonate like a melon idiocy," said enemies like Harlan Ellison, repeatedly. At night I was so stressed out with this problem I was too terrified to be alone. I used to sit quietly in the nursing station in the belief that the ultimate horror wouldn't happen in the company of others. Yet I did have friends. Once my head had been stuffed full of spore, it was miraculously and suddenly cleansed within a moment by someone I believed may have been Lord Jon Pertwee.

These were strange days. The Time Lords could experience increased grip on their skills when they drank black tea. Lord Jon sampled black tea from my own throat sometimes. His wife, who travelled under the name Sarah, directed me to make the drink in a special way without milk or sugar: A certain brew, a particular scent, traditionally squeezing the bag three times before dropping it. This tea energised them, sure, but it wasn't the way I usually took it. My grasp on the Gosfield Ward kettle was balanced between disliking the taste (saying I would never be sick for them) and abruptly making it when I was happy. But I was hardly ever happy. I only existed. *Vave-sims* and 'spore busters' assaulted me hand in hand through my incarceration, and the enemy took away my 'relief core'.

After years of my pineal gland being exacerbated by the enemy, giving my cigarettes a magnified affect, that month I discovered the dread contrast of blood-locks preventing the flow of nicotine through my body. They had called it a 'molecular key-hole', necessitating the short lived but hopeless want of a key for the lock. They also drove me berserk with nicotine 'matter-collectors' which was justified as "teaching me not to smoke" but that was blatantly back-to-front, because it made me want to smoke *more*. My blood stream was screaming for it and they piled on the 'guilt' such as suggesting an attack on Antimax with 'black (cigarette) tar'. At least that attack had been successful. A spacecraft dumped a shit-load of it over the lifeless planet, which tore itself to pieces. So did the spore assaults stop? No, Ellison made sure they continued; several times a day, everyday, for years and years.

I sought a God to worship for several weeks after the enemy destroyed my Christianity. They made me think that Jesus didn't understand, that He was flipping rude signs at me, and that He had made unfair laws about me long before. They made me think He was an alcoholic for wine fermented from the Holy Spirit, called *phase*-water, and they engineered a fear of prayer based on superstition about sincerity and spore death. I needed to feel cared for and loved from above. I worshipped each new God I was introduced to, but a terrible part of *vave-simulation* was when the Gods went wrong. It happened at least three times that year. I rarely attended church in my past but somewhere inside me I've always been a believer. This should help me find a path through the war, find love, and live through to a grand old age. If anyone hears me sneeze, if they say: "Bless you!" I reply, usually: "Someone's got to!"

CHAPTER TWENTY – <u>FEBRUARY: 1998</u>

Although I had exhibited much bravery during 1997 I had not believed that telepathy could kill anyone until the incontrovertible physical evidence of spore stress. I had nearly lost my life many times through murder simulation but the threat of spore in 1998 was a new and mortal terror. I didn't want my memories to disappear, or become misunderstood, so I was pleased to learn that there was a way for my experiences to become a testament above. A 'scune' could be used for purposes other than carrying possessions from *vicinity one* to Heaven. When moving my eyes from left to right along a horizontal line (such as the ceiling of a corridor) a *feelie* controlled 'scune' could absorb memories, at different speeds if necessary, so that by the day or the week I could update my record and have it all transferred up to the appropriate attending authorities.

In the 'set' I threw out all my tablets except *Zimmervane*. When I was caught I was re-prescribed medication "in liquid suspension", in a foul-tasting syrup. For a while I told the staff it was against my religion to swallow it with water and took a half-full carton of milk with me into the medication room. I would tip the beaker into my mouth and raise the carton, release the drug into the milk and pretend to swallow. Then I chucked the contaminated milk carton in the bin or poured it down the nearest drain. I may be one of the few in-patients who ever found a way of actually 'palming' syrup! I once raised a few smiles at medication time by comparing the drug trolley to a Dalek, saying "Exterminate, Exterminate!" I may not have been entirely joking. My answer to anyone caring enough to inquire how I was feeling was "just chugging along" like I was a yacht aspiring dignity struggling through sewage. My capabilities were stretched continuously by *vave-sims* of nonsensical realities.

On the level *above* everything I knew, our *Shield Dome* was the size of an egg. It was in an open box of others beneath the duress of the *Ton-u-lan* Ambassador, his partner and his four offspring. For no reason I could understand our universe was in this box, that was called a 'toning tray'. These creatures 'toned' any sphere getting too full of Quiddity by nullifying it. Although our dome was coated in silver Mythril and attention drawn to its sheen, it was located on the outer edge of the tray so out of reach of the four children: a Charlie, a Richard, a Clive, and a Sharlene. Their parents could destroy anyone with nullifying seats that may have been called 'Pav chairs'.

As a *Defender* of our dome, I rose and fought these creatures on their own heightened battlefield with the assistance of old Richard's soul, #108: Adrian Starliter – the "Angry Man". My advantage was that you don't have a lot to lose when using a *brick-through-self*. It can grip and walk and fight; yet it is diaphanous as a cobweb. The latent threat of spore hung over my skull like dark and unchanging cloud. Although I was literally tearing the spines out of the *Ton-u-lan* during the fight, we were nearing defeat: the moment when armed police officers arrived on the scene. They came down from the level above and secured the area with a sanity that seemed cheerful in comparison. They asked me if I wanted the *Ton-u-lan* Ambassador to be nullified in one of his own monstrous chairs. I had told the officer I didn't. The simulation returned to Earth.

The 'cyborg head' seemed to have more spore passing through its plates away from the hospital while I was treating myself to a new stereo system, in an electronics shop in Colchester, than at any other time. Or I seemed to notice it more poignantly then. I dealt with the sales-rep while porous venting clouds of the stuff with occasional flashes of dread.
I selected a solid twin component JVC, called a UX D88, which had excellent sound quality, and then they checked my bank details. I felt another flash of fear – this time of a fiscal nature – but I had forgotten I had arranged a legal £250 overdraft already! I packed the machine into a taxicab with a smile and was driven back to the ward. But I had skinned my 'stash' so close to the knuckle that I hadn't enough money left to pay the driver. So I pelted around the ward trying to borrow a few pounds that no one would lend

me. After all that excitement the bitch driver drove off with the machine and told me she would bring it back when I had the fare!

By the next afternoon I had set up the new stereo and it sounded beautiful. The strange thing about the Lakes, as I've said before, was that I felt strongly toward my little room. With its table and window and its sleepy bed, it was quiet, and 'home': it was *my room*: not my parents', *not* Thornfield Court, but my own place in which I felt safe in the micro-cosm of hospital life. I was watched over by two Alpha Centauri 'scor-polie', perfume ladies, law officers on a brick-down. They were responsible for the tracking and prevention of spore damage in their region. When I went to sleep the Time Lord Jon Pertwee arranged for porous venting each night at 2am. I made little noises at this time, so I was told.

After six weeks of spore assault I got assistance from old Richard's souls in countering possible damage. They came in, one at a time, to help with the making of a new 'power brain'. My favourite was Ricardo Mancianda, a friendly Spanish soul who had apparently led the life of 'Zorro'. During its creation I may have considered it a process of recovery but I also came to think that there could be more in it for me. As each new neural net was pasted in I realised I could end up with more abilities than those with which I had begun, maybe even overcome the alterations done to me by Barker when I was little. I could gain a tool for the processing of expression that truly befitted an artist and writer!

The essence of late 1997, that feeling of dying during sleep, was extended to the Lakes for a few days in the form of hundreds of black granules called 'REM pattern guns'. I walked around the hospital feeling like a zombie. The pellets were vicinity meshed with parts of the ward, sprinkled up the walls and over the floors, and they assaulted me with a lethargy so powerful it could burn and even knock out an old soul. Accepting I would die for a certainty one night I gave away the UX D88 and the crystal tortoise to different patients. I ordered a spore assault eat through different parts of my body to send up the *phase water* gradually but I woke up the next morning anyway. I got the stereo back but I never recovered the tortoise.

So, the '111 Power Brain' was my new grey matter. It had a wider focal area for assessing paintings (which most telepaths call the 'Whole Eye'); a deeper sensitivity of words; a podium stack of concentric circles of humour (stolen by a few comedians on a regular basis!) and other such interesting faculties. But apparently there were 'valves' in it. I never knew exactly what these were for but I guessed they were for the bypassing of caffeine and nicotine. When the valves were cleaned out the finished article was called the "111 (star) Power Brain". Feeling wrinkles forming flush with my skull, I had suddenly felt like painting but briefly because before the brain could be hardened with "rock form" rapture some bastard had sprinkled spore on the top of it and turned it to pulp. Since I believed everything I 'heard' I might not have realised then that my genuine antagonists were challenging me (and defending themselves) by engineering other enemies that didn't exist anywhere else except in my own perception. I had some genuine friends also, yet they were doing the same: psychoses, within psychosis.

One morning I came across Lord Zardak. That may have been his name. He was a fruit of the enemy initiative to rally higher forces to their flag by attracting allies through extending the distance of my broadcast telepathy. Lord Zardak heard it and came up the tunnel, in time, a long way from where his throne was suspended in The Big Bang. He brought with him an understanding of brains but perhaps had no grasp of who I was. His knowledge was the result of years of study: he commanded the rapture-tech to mould the human brain, to bend its processes to his will, but he had a lousy sense of what I was fighting for based in *vicinity one*.

His first rapture onto me was an insect brain that felt insane. Then he gave me a monkey's brain that was a relief after the insect but still hard to think with. Then, finally he gave me an ant brain through which it was impossible to have cogent thought – and I actually felt 'feelers' waving around on the top of my head! I replaced the throne at The Big Bang with two friends. I don't recall where Zardak ended up but I hope it involved celestial psychiatry.

I had stopped writing to Charlie Jordan. Not only because of the untenable horrors at the end of the year passed, but also because our souls were together now, and safe. During mid February I learnt of a lovely woman named Maddy Ashcroft. She was tall and slender with beautiful curly dark hair like Ruth Ann Regan of "All About Eve". Her first baby word had been "sun" and mine (being born four months before the successful Apollo 11 mission) had been "moon". She was an artist, a painter of trees. She deeply loved them and lived in a wooden house with a white picket fence on the edge of Hampstead Heath.

Maddy's soul had been hidden in oak trees for a long time until we could be together. And our time was coming. In comparison to those intervening years the waiting that remained was no time at all. I was falling for her, deeply, and it seemed to be our destiny to be together – in my first draft it is mentioned that I may have posted her letters. If this had even happened, which is doubtful, it must have been to an address I've since forgotten. When introduced to the idea of second woman, named Maddy Croft, I sensed a trap. This other was the 'croft of a non-smoker', a woman who's soul had been kept safe so long it had the taste of Bergundy wine. But Maddy Ashcroft was the first – the only Maddy for me – and I dismissed this other. Somehow a rogue Time Lord drank the wine anyway!

The 111 Power Brain had been hard come by. With my bank account being topped up and my very own assist – the "White Art" – those were aspects of what would become known as my "reward base". I checked my account regularly to see if the windfall had come in but one afternoon I received a gift of a nature far blacker than money, something growing from a speck in the 111. A creeping murder inflating

227

inside my skull that I was told was called "wyra tissue". I expected a cracked head for certain. When I was told the firing mechanism was "the sight of a ten pound note" I found that doubtful. The "wyra" became symbiotic with me, so I was still able to think through neural circuit adoption even when my brain had been completely taken over. And soon the thing started to talk! In a ponderous voice it wanted to know what was going to happen to it when it 'moved on' and a Time Lord came up with an answer: to rapture the wyra into a 'rabbit'. No doubt the rabbits had quite a horrible appearance – they looked like 'face-huggers' from the 1979 film *Alien* – but there were two, maybe three, made, and they could fly! The white wyra rabbit could painlessly inject a seed into the top of your head to tailor the growth of your own 111 Power Brain!

The best thing for me was the backache I had experienced on and off for over a decade was cured, cushioned as the tissue grew down my spinal column. It had never felt so comfy, so deliciously stretchable... The white rabbit flew about (disguised in grey sometimes?) and
I gathered about six telepaths had ordered rabbit seed to grow their own 111 Power Brains! They were taught wyra maintenance – I was told by my White Art. The tissue would stay healthy if you occasionally ate salty foods, like crisps; or rubbed a pinch of salt into the scalp. It was another one of those simulations intensified through physical verification. Since I couldn't hide the fact that I much preferred a "wyra" brain to a spore attack, the tissue faded.

The enticing belief in a financial reward due for my actions as a Defender was money that, as is typical of many people these days, I wanted to spend before I received it. So I returned to Thornfield Court in a cab looking for my old cheque book... found it; and armed with a £100 guarantee card, which had one of those shiny holograms on it, I thought: "let's go to town!" Where I had a lot of fun. In the space of three days I wrote twenty-two cheques and wound up a debt of over £1900! It was a mess of an account and even now, six years later, I'm still not allowed a guarantee card!

Other aspects of my Reward Base I drew up in the hospital's art room. Although I am not 100% certain that February was when it was written I would relate the contents anyway. As well as the 111, money, and assistance from the White Art, I wrote 'E'& 'T' about my relief-core. I would also wear the silver chain of a *Weaver* of my chosen art form; I would have a normal *reacher* and *verifier*, and a *language-reacher* (to communicate with birds and through which I had spoken to Alpha perfume ladies in late 1997), and I would have the capability of *Mirror Scrie.* When taking out a contact lens and macro focusing into the reflection of my own eye, there were 'visions' to be seen there, so I saw once. I seem to recall being advised not to *scrie* the future because allegedly it was the instrument of an occultist; but the skill seemed naughty and exciting to me, and I wanted it.

Another reward was the tool to allow me to write special books called *Nestrada* in which, later in life, I would describe the ideal heavens of aliens. And maybe – with a 'K' reacher imagination-drive – I would in some way actually help to engineer these heavens 'after' I had passed on. My knowledge of these races would be improved by visiting them in dreamt telepathy using a grand and special gift called the *R.E.M pattern Galactic Inter-lace!* During my first, I visited a nature conservation area on a Bark planet. I crossed a river and climbed a hillside where the aliens showed me a plant. It was laying eggs of creatures they called *Tortoi*, which had the appearance of tortoises that we have on Earth. Before I left the Barks gave me traditional clothing to try on: trousers and shirt of a rough but scintillating material in reds with gold thread. I woke up. That Barks were gay male creatures, as I had been told, was proved when I was informed they had watched me get undressed! Maddy and I were supposed to share another journey, a ride together with water entities on planets of solid water, called the Barvor. Galactic tourism from inside a submerged living creature – but sadly "I missed the train" because I didn't reach REM sleep in time.

The first *Nestrada* material I drew up was a heaven for mutated people called 'gimps'. No doubt a large part of me thought gimps were funny. They had become mutated (so I was told) by many generations continuous indulgence in tobacco. Their heaven had a three-story building for senior gimps, a golf course, ponies to ride, other little houses built into the side of a grassy hill like Hobbit holes, a club house and a pond. But one evening, sitting in the Gosfield ward smoking lounge, the writing of *Nestrada* became a much more serious issue. There were aliens watching. So I took notes.

The ideal heaven of the Barvor involved old country cottages like we have on Earth in *vicinity one* in gigantic revolving 'Air Stars', obviously the reverse to life in their worlds of water. One of them explained that the gravitational density at their planet's core was their 'hell'. Through my belief in re-incarnation I have thought in the past that there may not be any such place as 'hell'. Later on, a small Barvor asked me if the cigarette I was smoking was a "tookle" and was berated by a larger one for asking to sample it. I had thought this was a cute word, and after being told that 'tookle' were small highly addictive fish, the Barvor departed.

I had been imagining a tall slender woman come sweeping down the corridors of The Lakes: Maddy, in a flowing white dress like a cotton kite swirling in the darkness: proud in the act of rescue with an unquestionable dominance and beautiful in a way that sad place had never seen before. I had been writing to her on and off. And late one afternoon she said she was coming to Colchester. Maddy actually told me, with telepathy, that she was going to stay at the Riverside Hotel in North Station Road. So I planned my escape. I made sure that the door to the garden from the

Gosfield Ward smoking lounge was unlocked and put the two components of my UX D88 into a carrier bag. I dressed warmly and slipped into the darkness. At just past 11pm I started walking up Turner Road in the *opposite direction* to the Hotel to ensure I wasn't being 'tailed'. I left the stereo speakers in my wardrobe because I couldn't carry them, but if a member of staff saw them they might evoke the idea I would soon return.

Up the road, I phoned for a cab. My breath plumed like steam around the receiver. It was near freezing with a wind that was cold and black. The car dropped me near a gate that led to a path beside by the river. It was quiet and crisp, fresh. I stood for a moment on the grass watching two swans sleeping near the overhang of the bridge, floating with their beaks tucked under their wings. They mate for life I've been told. I observed them until I started shivering and then crept under an evergreen bush where I started stuffing handfuls of crunchy leaves up my jumper. Someone said it was an 'AS survival technique' but it didn't work. I recorded my 'scune'. Dawn wasn't for another seven hours, and after that Maddy would drive us to her house in Hampstead Heath. At some point in this adventure I was searched by the police. They found nothing illegal and drove away. Something had to be done to 'thaw me out' so I began collecting twigs and branches, scouring the ground in near blackness for dry fuel.

I built a bundle on the embankment by the water and used a short plank of wood as a break from direct heat. I put my lighter to it and soon it was ablaze. I backed up the path to check it wasn't visible from the road and saw it couldn't be seen for the trees and bushes. Larger sticks crackled, echoing to and fro in the flickering yellow light, as I lay on the bank with my boots near the river. I took out my tobacco pouch and made a hand-rolled cigarette shortly feeling as warm as newly toasted bread.

I drifted off into telepathic conversation with a beautiful feeling in my heart-box, which I was told was a "fire-box", a gift from the Lord who had encouraged the little blaze.

Maddy was on a 'live' *inter-lace* line while tucked up across the road. Her bed was less than 100 meters away and from it she may have muttered in her sleep that she was having a beautiful dream. Like the fire my gift heart-box would also be ash by morning, but I was to start a new life. Within hours of sunrise I would be looking out at the trees from Maddy's windows: her house, her secrets. I put the occasional branch on the fire, contented. I didn't notice the dewfall as blacks paled into shape with the typical greyness of an English February morn.

The light progressively brightened; the hand-fire was dying. I let it go. I stamped it out then walked past the place the swans had slept. Maddy said she would come across the road to the shop where I was buying stuff to eat for breakfast: yet she didn't. I knocked on the door of the hotel and went inside the seedy place with my heart-box disintegrating. The staff had no record of anybody staying with them with the name Ashcroft, or anyone fitting Maddy's description. She hadn't even stayed, as some telepath had suggested, in the plusher setting of The George Hotel up the hill on the High Street. She had never been in Colchester at all.

My chest felt tired. I was tired, swaying in pain at a bus stop with the stereo feeling heavy in its bag. I had been let down by women in Ireland, Clacton, London, and now – in my own hometown… yet the tenderness survived. I rode a tall bus on the top deck of a ticket back to the hospital. Maddy might have called it a test of my commitment, of my love, of courage in my escape. I didn't want to lose her. I couldn't live this thing out alone in a war in which I was mostly just a victim for long without someone to call 'girlfriend'. Yet, for now, we were together. Back in my room at the hospital I patched the stereo back together and climbed under my covers. I bid Maddy goodnight.

CHAPTER TWENTY-ONE – <u>MARCH: 1998</u> *Hospital six*

Knowing the fruit that symbolised *The Art* I didn't eat an apple for six months. 1997 had passed me by in a hideous blur yet I recalled it as being an 'adventure', a generalisation, a typical defence mechanism of our minds through which most nastiness is erased. 1998 was made of different terrors. I was making tea one afternoon and I exhibited psychological damage when I started crying over the kettle. I had been fighting continuously and hard for twelve months, and the stark comparison to the teapot in my mind; symbolic of happiness, clean living, and simple pleasures... it broke through the dam I had built to protect my inner emotional self. The experiences of war on the front-line, the fear perceived and the terrible things seen and done, can affect soldiers for life. I cried like something had been stolen but I quickly had to mend the chinks in my armour because that is how I continued, adapted, survived. In a conflict where no soft targets are left alone you can't walk around wearing your heart on the outside.

Since when I lay with Heather I felt it would be pleasant to smoke with a partner after making love, wanting *feelie* life to reflect *vicinity one*, so the feelie-sticks moved to front stage. It is unlikely that I introduced these to the Starion Plains, alone. Cigarettes have been around for over a hundred years but the issue of addiction became a larger part of the war. *Vave-sims* of this kind had me banging my head against wooden doors and mirrors with frustration. I could see the danger coming and I knew it needed to be regulated so I constructed the Gold Stick Police. It was a good idea but nevertheless it never took off *because* it was a good idea.

Other Time Lords came into vogue: half a reconciled Dalek called Davros, Tom Baker, and other men that had played the role of 'The Doctor'. I lit up a cigarette in the Gosfield Ward kitchen, once, and something happened that would affect me for many months. The leader of the Time Lords was attending, perhaps because I was making tea, but part of him was curious and tempted to sample the cigarette. He did so and it was a knee-jerk reaction to reject his instantly nicotine addicted personality, splitting into two entities: the goodness of the tea drinking Lord Jon Pertwee; and the other half bad and black, called Jon Pertwee's Soul. Initially I feared the second had taken all the time-turning capabilities but events later disproved that.

Needless to say I strived to protect my loved one. Defending Maddy was some of the most stressful experiences of those days. Her *scu* had become a target, for Harlan Ellison, for the bloody knives and saws and cleavers of his monstrous 'chop centres'. Since she had told me she had been suffering nightmares for years I didn't want her pain to be compounded by that sadist memory-returning his victims back again and again. This memoir is itself full of horrors, but the things I was brought to believe Ellison did then are too disgusting and frightful to include in this writing. I used to go crazy when she was attacked like that. With the well-being of the both of us at stake I hid her *scu body* in protective vicinities called "cuddle-stones", crystals inside which her *scu* could attain safety and softness on a *brick-down,* with a mutual sigh of relief.

The daily grind of the 'set' continued: Palming medication, the lockout of caffeine from my blood stream, the bladder trouble and the harassment about smoking: the potentially lethal assault with spore everyday, the wyra tissue and the long slow sweep of the minute hand of the clock, ticking; the nightmares, and the *vave-sims*. "Worlds within worlds" Barker had written. And I learned of some of them: *Tarterous* with its sadistic 'cenobites', a hell of bizarrely body-pierced demons illuminated about their strange deeds by a blue light in a place of swirling dust and gore. And Gehenna, a place of classic hell-fire and brimstone ruled by a sexless creature called The Thrall, which swayed like a shit pile with arms and legs everywhere, yet soon to become undismissible.

Verbalizing both sides of a conversation out aloud I was increasingly drawing the attention of the nursing staff. At my quietest I was spore-stressed. At other times I could get angry, shouting about blood-locks and 'matter-collectors', but I never got into a rage – sometimes I pandered. Often I was pushed around by the Cusper regiment, of which here is new detail: In Barker's 'back pocket box' I believed these water Qualm and air Qualm aliens were each 100 feet tall, a rank and file army centralized on Asgaroth circles called the 'Cusper Po'. There was a metal plate of vacuous 'back-time' behind my heart-box, which was meshed with a dustbin on the Cusper Po into which they tossed bits and pieces of trash, and sometimes people's *subtle bodies*. How many of them actually deserved it should be considered in conjunction with a magazine that was new out that month called: "The Nullility Escape Journal Issue #1" Maybe my antagonists had more friends and I had more enemies than I had previously realized. Beneficial credibility can come in swings and roundabouts.

I have never suffered the extreme ups and downs of bi-polar depression yet in those days I experienced genuine happiness for only brief moments. The pain of destroyed naivety (like Stamp's horror dreams being called "Happy Times") caused a sadness in me that had to be buried, about which I never got angry. Subconsciously fearful of loveliness being hurt I reacted to my life's contrast to such beauty very often with confusion and less often with tears, about which the enemy used to say: "Let's see a big tear roll down his cheek" But I found true rage, like many patients, at the moments I was most misunderstood and mistreated.

Kneeling in the garden, by an ornamental well, I heard a nuclear device had blown up in Washington. I started yelling. The Pentagon was gone, blown away like a sandcastle in a hurricane, and the future was now bleak and terrible. I was crying, and was suddenly surrounded by five or six staff that had burst into the garden. Not compressing the rage I was experiencing they half-carried me back into the ward, kicking and screaming; dragged me into a room with no furniture and a piss-proof mattress and stuck me with needles. I recovered my breath... and soon I was beginning to drift, and to nowhere that was any good.

It is an irony of the mental health system that patients who always get angry are violently smothered while there are therapy groups called "Getting In Touch With Anger" for people that never do. In the restraint room I started hallucinating *intenseiform*. I was floating towards the nose bones of a skull and I knew it was going to be a 'bad one' as I entered the twin holes of its nostrils. I found myself in a place that I believed heroin addicts go to teach them a dire warning. Most of it I can't remember but I was sinking, in there, and saw images of bizarre executions. Not fully conscious I don't remember when the staff let me out, but I couldn't have been in the room for long. I had wanted to stay awake to beat the sedation, but I fell asleep. Anything would have been preferable to hallucinating that stuff with my eyes open.

I was now on Section Three of the Mental Health Act: Six months of involuntary treatment since about 25th January. One of the drugs I had been 'coshed' with was *Acuphase*, the first of three injections administered every three days. It was powerful enough to make a flea out of an elephant and I hated it. Had I known this was to be a nine-day course of the drug I could have prepared, somehow, but preparation wouldn't have stopped me hating it. Dose #2 was brought into my room beside the nursing station at about 9:30 in the morning. The staff woke me up with a needle that looked bio-hazardous and rude in a metal kidney dish. I may have got angry but I don't remember if I was restrained. It doesn't seem likely that the staff would take a patient directly from sleeping in his bed to the restraint room. I should have taken it standing up and gone back to sleep, but I was developing a reputation for losing control.

I was interviewed by two staff from a tougher hospital, in the Colchester area, called Willow House. They had made a locked-unit out of an entire floor, but... how long is a piece of string? I managed to 'blag' my way out of being admitted but

I got into a fight with a new patient in Gosfield Ward smoking lounge. I said heroine was a bad deal and the offended man had come at me suddenly, and hard. The staff broke us apart. Being inept at melee in *vicinity-one* I was surprised to hear that he had reported a fear of me to the staff.

I was in a different bedroom in the process of recovering from the tail end of the second jab. I was feeling 'better in myself', a psychiatric colloquialism, but like the myth of the man who had to push huge rocks up a hillside and always lost his stamina near the top – so the staff crashed in on my privacy with another needle and the rocks fell back down. I didn't want to go back to that ghostly existence. When I saw the syringe being picked out of its obscene shiny dish I climbed up onto the end of the bed, and started kicking and spitting at them. My back was against the wall, literally and metaphorically. I hated them but I couldn't prevent getting a stab below the hip, and then they left me to it. I drifted. It was one of the last days I was on Gosfield Ward for many weeks. I soon had to pack my things because I was being transferred to a higher security unit. Small things, like my oil paint box, camera, clothes and boots, quality pens, the tape and C.D. Walkmans with speakers and some discs, mostly purchased during the cheque-book binge. The big stereo was left behind to be secured by my parents. I was taken to North London.

The ambulance dropped me off at a private I.C.U, in Walthamstow, called Abbeydale Court. I was taken through the double 'airlock configuration' entrance doors, both most likely made of reinforced glass, and then was immediately put into a restraint room while I was processed.

I could see through the window that, as my baggage was searched, much of it was being strewn about on the floor around the nurse's station. I was cowed, I called them all 'sir', and realised, that in comparison to Abbeydale Court, The Lakes had been a like a session of mini-golf. This place was a prison.

During the day there were <u>at least</u> four staff on duty, most all of them black or Asian. The main corridor from the nurse's station passes the TV room. It zigzags diagonally past the patients' doors, up to a staff-room by the smoking lounge. There are <u>two restraint rooms</u> for seven bedrooms... warm and stuffy, all the windows on the ward are sealed and cannot be unlocked for air. Your own bedroom door is a feeble barrier. The only true privacy available was when I was splashing about in the en-suite bathroom. The smoking lounge had a view of the back of a wooden fence with a door in it, which I used to wonder about. Trees were rising above it, a forest there. Could the door be unlocked? In Abbeydale Court any leave that was taken outside, started at five minutes by the back-fence, was called *parole*.

Although the smoking lounge was the social centre of the ward you weren't allowed to keep your own lighter. You don't appreciate such a thing until it's gone and you could only get alight from the staff. There were a few armchairs in the room and a battery-powered stereo padlocked to the wall. Like the television set the stereo was switched off at midnight. Caffeine relief could only be had three or four times per day. As we couldn't brew tea or coffee for ourselves we were usually dribbling mad for it, and slurped several cups each. Visitors had to be observed by a member of staff in the dining room. That was where I celebrated my 29th birthday, 12th March 1998.

I met my parents across a table, and they gave me some presents. I don't remember what all of them were but I was allowed to walk with them down to the shops. I nudged Dad into buying me a pack or two of luxury cigs and fifty grams of Golden Virginia. Under the tight fitting lid of the container was a heavy weight of moist tobacco, protected by foil leaves, and I used to call it my *Magic Tin*. I was too organised to run out. That was one of the reasons a nurse regularly went to the shops, for us, because if none of us had anything to smoke a riot could have ensued!

Long after the Gold Stick Police were dispersed the way was paved for more guilt related *vave-simulation* about smoking. Small deyaforms started sucking my blood stream dry like I was a fuel pump: absorbing, packaging; *feelies* collecting sticks that dropped out of their fix-machines, trading in sticky brown lumps of the stuff for the 'cash' of Starion Plain's credits.

S*cu* in my inner vicinity captured nicotine in horizontal plates in my chest made of a subtle material that they harvested like honeycomb. They 'smoked' when I did, using sacks flush with my ribs called "lung bags", often engineered smaller than mine for a suffocating affect. I was inflicted with poisons that were a sickening reverse, perhaps, of my favourite essences called "tea-la-la" and "cig-la-la", and the Gehennan's had their own "nescrose" to smoke, which to almost everyone else was a poison also. In spite of being a living person who had not broken any material plain laws I was presented as the 'source' of this trouble. Sometimes I was *matter-collected* to smoke more, but the 'hunger striker's breakfast', that relaxing feeling of a tea and cigarette 'combined molecule' was gone. And something had to be done about it.

There was a Barker soul on the plains, apparently on the side of good, named Clive Bactu, meaning "Back to God". I believed he was doing useful raptures but then discovered he had been producing fix-machines. After I had exposed what Barker the man had done to me and revealed his false mythology I had felt victory so I found two places for his soul to be put out of harm's way. One offer was to become a musical note that I had read about in an "Alfred Hitchcock and the Three Investigators" book under the covers when I was at school, a kind of 'reward for evil', a subsonic bass note that is almost undetectable to the human ear but the vibration of which instils an uneasy fear in people.

And the other idea was to put him into a locked universal unit: an Asgaroth of nullility with paper, a pen, a cubula, and twenty feelie-sticks per day, and guarded by at least 7000 Gold Stick Police. The idea of incarceration on such a gigantic scale was perhaps considered ridiculous and lessened to that of a smaller, galactic, plate. I heard he soon started writing a book called "1001 Ways to Kill Richard". The police force I had arranged to guard him was, as I have reported, disbanded, and his galactic prison was forced out of my thoughts. The facts presented in that *sim* had been gradually changed, on a long and subtle time-line; in other words cancelled.

After experiencing new things through synchronicity, indicating the existence of a higher force, co-incidences *talking* to you directly... well, then, like myself, you may say that nothing surprises you anymore. I believed Lord 'K' to be the Asgaroth of the Earth. He looked after our weather, held us safe in our orbit, and I believed that his wife was the very Deyaform that rotated us. But like the *feelie* of my old boss in London during '91, who had presented himself as God after dying of lung cancer and evolved into some kind of nicotine insane 'demon' that only Tarteran cenobites could restrain. In another *vave-sim* I was forced into thinking that Lord 'K' was the monster Barker's brother. Yet again, I must have believed that I had lost a God to pray to. But I kept looking.

In the hospital dining room, there was a drum of chilled mineral water. Cooling my throat with a cupful, I felt an awareness of doing well. There was a purity about water that was appealing to me, religiously. I used to go to sleep holding a cold bath towel in my arms like it was a baby, the towel I dried off with after one of my other pleasures, 'Water Festivals'. These began with a shocking cold shower to refresh everywhere; the steel sink filled to overflowing with freezing water, splashing about on the bathroom floor, and heaving great handfuls of it all over myself. When I had dried off I experienced a pleasurable clean glow in my inner spirit that I was told was called *dopamine X / Y*. I used so much water in these festivals that it crept under the wall of my bathroom and soaked the corridor carpet on the other side!

The *feelie* soul of a dead Alpha Centauri 'perfume lady' is a spirit creature that was called a "Water Fe". They looked like manta rays and 'swim' like graceful birds with a little stalk on their heads called a 'feeler frond'. I gathered that there were Fe high up on our own Earth (Starion) Plains, also. Their delicate 'feeler fronds' could transfer morsels of food between vicinities. I used to unwrap little Babybell cheeses and crunch sour cream and onion Pringles, and they would sample tiny crumbs of it from my own mouth. Their visits almost had the essence of feeding fluffs of bread to baby birds. In their purity, apparently representatives of water, I felt I might be able to pray to them and I was introduced to a Fe that was close to me already, closer than I could have realized.

Crofty and I learned that our daughters would be called Joy and Bethelay, if we wanted them to be so named, and that they would actually have *feelies* originating from two Water Fe, *of Alpha Centauri!* The proximity of a 'grand plan' about this was daunting and nearly beyond my grasp, but I knew it was special. I learned I had been praying to a Water Fe goddess that was actually going to become my own daughter! This didn't really work in my position on religion. I didn't want the one to whom I prayed to, to speak back. After so many months of hearing 'voices' quietness is, needless to say, a large part of what I still seek. That and love.

In Walthamstow I had a couple of experiences in the bathroom that had a lot more impact than a 'Water Festival'. One night it seemed to be the safest place to hide from a rocket-propelled-grenade. These two telepath men, looking down the barrel of their launcher at the hospital, needed talking to. I can't remember what we discussed but I talked them out of it. They went away. On another occasion, I found myself pushed into a gigantic *brick-through* where I discovered *Hellraiser* puzzle boxes called 'Gorkons'. Hell that existed 'outside' the skin of that reality model. I cracked open four of them and hundreds of thousands of souls were freed who found relief in vicinities that were the opposite of where they had been. Some were absorbed into the soft weave of 'Fred' and some went into cold water; some went into a box of chocolates and others were honoured to take places in the electrical segments of Lord 'K's Earth Asgaroth.

The correct choices in destiny began in Walthamstow. Maddy and I would eventually meet. I knew this. In spite of her mortal enemy Regan Capshaw: 'alien dream-attack system', cult leader and caster of nightmares, Regan would not prevent Maddy becoming my fiancé who, from now on, I will call Crofty. I was relaxed in the certainty of our future. Until one night I saw an actor on TV that looked like a killer. He inspired dread in the mere fact of his existence. He was actually out-there, somewhere, and instantly swept into the simulation as the *Genetic Corer*. He entered the war through the connection I shared in Crofty's life: the 'theatre' of the *live-interlace* line. I learned that this killer could cancel our destiny, so the certainty was gone, but not so far that I would go down without a fight.

I was already safe. No one without approval could enter or leave the unit. The battle for Crofty's life began shortly after I had been sexually teasing her *scu*. I hadn't known that her physical self was sleeping in a hole in the ground aiding some friends of hers, activists defending some green belt scheduled to be overcome by a motorway. She awoke with the cool musky scent of earth in her nostrils to be told the Law was forming up in riot gear. It was to be the final day of the protest. The policemen had their visors down and were standing in a faceless line clacking batons against their shields. The blues were going to beat the greens hands-down. Everybody knew it – and Crofty was standing between the Law and the land, at the front.

The riot police began to advance. The situation was looking dangerous so I yelled "Back off Maddy! Get the hell out of there!" and she did. She escaped in a car heading to one of the Shires with some friends. They drove into the afternoon to an abandoned property that was their dream: a derelict manor house that they wanted to fashion into a commune for homeless activists to call home. But they were followed.

Telepath Regan Capshaw (who I was obviously confusing with Ruth Ann Regan) and her cult were closing in. Her boyfriend Patrick Tilley and their psychopathic disciples parked at the top of the driveway. In the light of the disappearing sun, armed with mostly wooden and blade weapons, some carrying red canisters of petrol, they were spoiling for a fight and walked down the path. I managed to keep in *inter-lace* contact with Crofty. If my loved one was hurt I would know about it the instant she did. On my 'live' link the two sides were actually converging, for real, and the green friends were out-numbered. They fought but by the end the battle was won by fire. Crofty escaped intact, ahead of Capshaw, but their dream home was an inferno. The burning lit up the land for miles around and everyone fled in fear of it attracting the authorities. With it many of Crofty's hopes were charring into yearnings. Herself and an old friend left the Shire for Colchester by car, and there I guided them up to Thornfield Court, a place I knew well enough to make a stand. Most telepaths knew the address of that flat. The year before I had believed that cars driven by enemies on their way to Colchester had been blown off the A12, by the wind of Lord 'K', at least twice!

Capshaw increased her reception and put her mind out like a sonar-array. Many of her crazed followers were still with her. The 'Y' balcony was the only way to the top floor, the only access in or out of Flat 12. I must have guided Crofty to a door key that was hidden outside under a flowerpot. Near to it was standing my blue Honda CG125 motorcycle. Although even a small car couldn't fit the paths that led to the foyer, the bike could navigate the garden paths easily as I had done many times myself. It might make an ideal reserve escape vehicle. By the time Crofty learnt how to use the handles and gears to drive it, Capshaw was forty minutes closer to the flat. They were coming and they were armed, far crazier than most of the mentally ill people I had met over the years. We needed to construct defences.

Crofty's driver had been a neighbour of hers. If I remember rightly, he'd had a crush on her for years. On my suggestion they started looking for wood to protect their position from 'missiles' coming through the windows (stones at best, and at worst Molotovs) but they couldn't find any. I don't know whether the phone had been connected but calling the police occurred to none of us. I waited, within my woman during the calm, then came the noises of car doors slamming and the voices of people on the paths. The cultists had arrived, and brought with them the deadly bubble of a lynch-mob mentality. Crofty's friend went down to meet them. He went down alone: a brave man.

He met them halfway between the road and the 'Y' floor. Tilley was standing at the head of the rabble holding a gun and threatened Crofty's friend to "stand aside". The man charged at Tilley instead, making a grab for the weapon, which fired with a noisy flash…then it all became quiet. It was Tilley that crumpled up. The mob's leader's boyfriend lay bleeding over the cement and reality gate-crashed the cultist's bubble. I told Crofty to mount the motorcycle. She started it and drove it outside. I assumed her brave friend was going to be all right on his own. He didn't get into his car or ride pillion with her, maybe because this would have threatened the impasse.

She rode through the cultists with deliberation who parted before her in a kind of group concussion, like the sea before Moses. She turned onto the Fingringhoe Road and headed for another place I knew well, Mersea Island. It was about fourteen miles away. When she arrived, she rode to the Esplanade and hid beneath a beach hut as two (telepath?) policemen walked passed her on the sand just feet from her head. Maddy wasn't a *feelie*, or a *scu*, or a fundament; she was flesh and blood, sexy at that, and she had a heart that beat for us both. When the police were gone I realized she needed a warm bed for the night. I didn't want her to be cold so I advised her to ride back to Colchester and get a late train to London. She had friends at her place in Hampstead Heath. She re-mounted the machine and its headlamp led her primitively through the night to North Station where she purchased a ticket to London.

Once she was sitting happily onboard, clacking and clattacking along the rails to Liverpool Street, there was another impasse – this one of my own: I could relax. It was possible Capshaw's cult had disintegrated. Crofty was comfortable and warm and safe. In the past Capshaw hadn't attacked her all the time, wherever she went, so I assumed (in my original handwritten version) that this might have been because Crofty used a kind of cloaking device
called a 'telepathy blanket', thus perhaps screening herself from the dreaded *Genetic Corer* also. Made of a visualised dimension three ('K' material made solid) some telepath women use such a blanket when taking their ablutions.

She got a cab from the station to the edge of the forest. Safely indoors, she had a shower while her friends made her some hot tea and something to eat. Her home virtually didn't exist officially because of her celebrity. But there was another place she could seek that offered total protection: a mental health ward. In a secure unit she would be unreachable. She might have acted on it; Crofty was very tired... The Corer's attack happened *before* she got ready for bed – and perhaps *after* she had telephoned

Hammersmith Hospital to volunteer for treatment. The *Genetic Corer* was coming in. Armed, and without a mask, logically because he didn't think anyone in the house would survive to make his description.

There was a silencer screwed into the end of the barrel and he opened fire on her friends. The pistol made coughing noises as it dropped empty cartridges onto the steps, wisps of cordite filled the air as he mounted the stairs. Crofty's friends were knocked off their feet. She had never got ready for bed so she could at least make an escape bid without wasting time having to get dressed. She climbed out of an upstairs window and slid down the red tiles and dropped to the earth. She looked back at her house and saw the beginnings of dreadful flickering light. The wood was soon burning with a hunger familiar to her tired eyes. She turned her back on it. Once again Maddy Ashcroft was out in the cold and had lost another home to fire. Although admittance is usually done via a referral from a G.P., the staff on the ward in Hammersmith took her in that same night. In spite of wearing clean clothing she didn't have to act. It was obvious to them she was in genuine distress. She was cold, scraped, exhausted, and terrified. They led her to a bed she had been given on the ground floor. There were nice clean sheets on it, perhaps a duvet, and a tablet. She went to sleep. I went to off to bed myself but getting to sleep may have taken me longer.

The rules at Abbeydale Court, with its coffee break-to-coffee break routine, the smoking and the bullshit food, institutionalised patients quickly. Things were stolen often. I lost two silk shirts, some walking boots, a Walkman and a roll-film camera to theft. There was a couple of black men 'at court' and the stereo in the smoking lounge played mostly rap. One man was silent and wore the blue wardrobe of a gangster, and the other was a young Muslim who had such a talent for 'street poetry' I gave him a luxury pen as encouragement. I was smoking more roll-ups in that 'set' for a longer time than ever, developing a yellow stain on my right fingertips that I called a 'fighting scar'.

There were actually *two* Starion Plains: the Upper was for genuine *feelies*, and the Lower was for addicts and dealers that ran around burning each other with 'pav guns' like it was the Wild West or something. Below was Stargore (a bloody mess of past-policy Ellisons) Tarterous, and Gehenna – whose leader The Thrall had made his Hell into a kind of social club. The Gehennans used to creep about in the middle of the night, climb up onto the Asgaroths of the Lower Plains with vacuum cleaners where they hoovered up the butts of feelie-sticks. They took them back down to use in making *Nescrose*. Yet none of these realities seemed as real to me as the *live-interlace line* with Madelein.

The next day I encouraged her to get a room upstairs in the hospital. She was scared and told the staff she wasn't safe on the ground floor. She wouldn't have let go the address of the second fire but her desire for forty feet between herself and the ground that the Genetic Corer walked upon probably looked like a certain case of paranoia. But they did move her, and two days went by. I do not remember if I showed her how to 'palm' her medication at this time. Perhaps it had been a good intention that was never realised but I would have recommended she keep *Zimmervane,* if she could get it, because I believed it could instil 'dark sleep', in new users, that it could induce a virtual dreamlessness that might beat Capshaw's 'nightmaring'. We were relaxed in our similar environments. I started to work out a romantic possibility that Crofty be transferred to Walthamstow. We could meet one another in Abbeydale Court and get locked up together in bullet-proof bliss! So the posts were moved forward. An inter-hospital referral would instil a joy that could snap Clive Barker and win the war. But it never happened. I never met her because on the second night the security of the first floor at Hammersmith was fatally compromised.

The quietness and the dim night lighting of the place was sleepy but exploded with noise. Glass shattered over the fire escapes as masked men exploded through the first floor windows, guns fired, deafening. Bullets raked the beds with thumps of small feathers and the clattering echoed through corridors, muzzle flashes and screams. I was connected to Crofty in mutual terror. Most of the people running about were to find no escape. Some patients never knew it end, and many of the staff trying to assist them were shot off their feet; then

CROFTY WAS DOWN! She was struck in the left thigh! The killers faded like gun smoke in the drafts through the broken windows, and Crofty was carried down on a stretcher. I didn't know if the wound had rent a major artery. That was my reality. If they could get her into the ambulance quickly enough for the paramedics to do their work, then she may be saved. When she was inside the vehicle, on the bunk, I dared to breathe again... but this story was to reach closure in the worst way. The man in the back of the ambulance with her was the *Genetic Corer*. There was nothing I could do to prevent it. He sawed her leg off and she died quickly. Crofty was gone.

I was asked later if I wanted to die myself and was offered a 'cusper heart-cannon', a spiked mechanical device *vicinity-meshed* with the left-hand heart of a fundament. I was fed up, tired of the spore, and tired of trials in the material plane that on retrospect had been a slog. Dropping the whole thing and going to Heaven to be with Crofty was appealing, so I accepted the 'heart-cannon' and every spasm in my chest was bringing us closer together. That night there was a lustreless attempt at marrying our souls. It didn't occur to me to wonder what Charlie's *feelie* was supposed to do in this position. I didn't think about her at all. But I have believed that sometimes a person can non-consciously construct *more than one soul* in a lifetime. The ceremony didn't satisfy me anyway. I slept.

The next afternoon an entity asked me if I wanted to live. Perhaps this question was also a question of the strength of my resolve, yet I had exhibited the commitment to take a heavenly place with a woman's *feelie* soul before. Crofty had returned to the trees she so loved, so I was told... and so I said "yes", I said "*life*" and it was done. The trauma faded like bubbles on the surface being the only evidence of a ship that had sunk, a ship that could have been named "The Worst Vave-Simulation Ever" that had vanished to the bottom of a cold grey sea and would never be seen again.

As a receiver of 'voices' I have spoken the truth virtually continuously since the very beginning and I write the word 'virtually' to avoid the possibility of lying. I like facts but sometimes it feels like I don't come across such certainties very often. Expressing the truth of facts can feel awkward since I have been questioned and spore assaulted simultaneously whatever my answer. You already know I write words such as 'probably' and 'maybe' and

'perhaps', which you may feel are inaccuracies, but for me they actually *add* accuracy. Except for sometimes teasing the enemy I have told the truth since the early days sensing that a lie would stick out like a sore thumb. Inner *scu* have called me 'transparent' in the past. In my quest I have generally sucked up the bullshit like a man starving for vitamin 'C' sucking up plump grapes: the whole bagful regardless of quality - and assimilated my discoveries in my search for the truth. The truth is something even liars want!

The truth is almost always more important when you don't have it, like FBI agent Fox Mulder
in The 'X' Files, who searches for it everywhere. The expression THE TRUTH IS OUT THERE on the last page of the show's title sequence has at least two meanings. "The truth is <u>out there</u>", can mean out in the world, geographically, or "The truth is *out there*" can also mean that it is 'out there' – like it's crazy. *Two truths,* which are a matter of the viewer's individual perception as in the case of a telepath's

white or black 'K' viewpoint. I've had a rapture blade called the *Knife of Gurion* stuck in my back a few times in 1997 that allegedly engaged black 'K' and on the night mentioned on page 75 I really went through the wringer. On that same page, I also wrote up: 'The Sword Of Truth Is Sharper Than A Lie'. After nearly a lifetime of 'driven thinking' and fourteen years since I was first admitted onto a psychiatric ward, I am now starting to experience more of my own thinking. More thoughts that are actually mine - and that *IS* good!

The dread Dimension Two of the *Helter Incendo* if moulded under Rapture could be made to feel amusing. A telepath with 'a dimension #2 Bone Of Hue' in their rib cage finds just about anything they encounter hilarious. 'Hue' is an abbreviation of 'Humour'. I had a 'bone' of my own in 1997. In Walthamstow I discovered that a man I admire, Premier Tony Blair, had been given (by Barker?) a 'Dimension #2 <u>Banana</u> Of Hue' for his joking and chuckles. But the material could seep into the skeleton, and thence perhaps into the mind. Some telepaths had been worried about his dreams… but, far be it than me to get between a man and his banana; he didn't want to lose his funnies. Yet an answer was found – to make one out of Quiddity material - a *Quiddiere* Bone of Hue to replace his dangerously virile banana. Hmmm. I suppose the whole thing could have been a *Vave-Simulation*. If all our mobile phones had vave-sim cards instead of sim-cards the phone company would still make a fortune but there wouldn't be any real people to talk to.

When my psychiatrist saw me at Review I did a lot of acting and she believed I was recovering. I remember thinking to myself that I agreed, to some extent, but why was I feeling better without taking medication? I doubted I would have felt so good if I had actually taken the stuff and that casts the whole psychiatric thing in a poor light. She wrote me up for some genuine parole: twenty-five minutes in the forest! If I had died of that heart cannon, because of an invented situation, then the vave-simulation would have ended with me and its engineers would have been in a shit-load of trouble - and that's the likely reason they gave me a chance at life. But the simulations never really ended. As long as I was naïve and deluded enough for them to be my preferred reality they just continued to evolve, and some went on for so long that they might have become another kind of reality also - for those that made them.

I spent time in the forest accompanied by a nurse. They usually waited at a discrete distance while I revered Crofty's memory. It was spring. The new growth adorning the trees was delicate in colour and texture. It was cool and fresh under the thin canopy, and I placed offerings into a bole cupped between two roots at the base of an old tree. It may have been an oak. I placed things in there to Crofty's spirit, like feathers and stones and interesting bits of wood. I would talk to her; perhaps she heard.

Soon my grief lost its edge and I was introduced to a telepath of Royalty, a lady that shared her Christian name with my late Maddy. I entered into new relations: with Princess Madelein Lamarkristen of the Hungarian Royal Family! She was perhaps nice, pretty in her way. I showed her my body in the bathroom mirror and started to grow a beard. We made plans like building a tree house in an ancient oak: One room with a large bed, and a glass ceiling through which to gaze at the stars. But best of all <u>she was safe</u>, she was enclosed in an environment with tall guards and taller walls. I was 'low-born', so having a problem with British Royalty. It was troubling but I felt my relationship with the princess should go ahead if possible. I was also involved with other vicinities, heard that my old soul from 1997, named "Boo" (Charlie's nickname for "Bune") had got into trouble in Gehenna - so I went down there to investigate. I was back in the fight!

Using a *brick-through self* I discovered Boo locked in a room cowering under a table. The bastards had been cutting off his skin, preparing it in a drum, and aerating the mixture through a *feelie* stick to manufacture nescrose. So I attacked the place with dimension three grenades, and a couple of relatively harmless 'nuclear devices' but with a familiar feeling of helplessness, because of 'memory return'. It was not always a defensive measure. In Stargore they used it on *remriece beds* to repeat tortures and revive victims. It turned out that Boo was lucky in the way he was eventually rescued. Since I cared, so was I. A giant hand had come down called a "Spiritual Ambulance" which had helped me before and it came down with fingers about six feet long, plucked up Boo and took him up to the Lower Plains. I chilled out with a cigarette in the company of a small bearded man, the quiet gentleman of the lounge, a friend called Gary.

Gary must have witnessed some of my conflict. The talking aloud with the strutting about, and the wild gestures; the appearance of a man insane, but he never asked me about it. Neither did another patient rumoured to have played drums with a famous band. Our confidences were probably shallow but a pleasing respite from telepathy. We used to play CDs on my portable stereo and I was Gary's hero when I managed to recover one of my lighters from the contraband envelope so we could light our own cigarettes. On another occasion we started transferring our hot drinks to the smoking lounge during coffee breaks. We used plastic cups cadged from the water dispenser and most staff grudgingly allowed this practise. Even with my detested blood-locks the tea and nicotine could still mix a little in my brain. It was better than nothing. We had manipulated weaknesses in the system and were much happier!

Barker told telepaths that if he were killed 'time would stop'. I don't think I believed him but I did believe in a *live interlace* with a man who was hunting him down. Barker was making some of his fans into 'decoys'. If he needed them he 'shouted' to be invited in, filled them with Dimensions Two, then used them as platforms from which to continue operating anonymously. On the *interlace* line the hunter caught up with Barker in an industrial area like docklands, with a firearm. He shot Barker many time at close range. The body was impossibly animated; rolling about, spitting and writhing long after a normal body would be dead. The cause was concluded to have been Rapture, and of the blackest kind.

The enemy used 'attack-spore' everyday of the week. It was inter-dimensionally pumped along a pipe called a 'nose bow' through my nostrils and to inflate the inside my head. A nearby galactic 'plate' of robots attacked me like this a lot. Air carried spore 'sub-drives' had once killed everyone in the world in eleven and a half hours. The dreadful sensation, which Ellison spoke about with the essence of a car crashing into sewage, was a horror that came from questioning the integrity of my skull. In The Lakes the Asgaroth of that robot galactic went on and on and on in a litany of increasing spore sizes and dividing speeds. I discovered that their leader was Slarti Bartfast (of *Hitch Hiker's Guide* fame) but even knowing that, there was little I could do about it. In the past Lord Jon had assisted with spore venting in the middle of the night and it was good having that kind of support. There were most likely others backing me up whose names I didn't know.

The Time Lords scooted around vicinities in a pair of old English police telephone-boxes traditionally called TARDIS's. The good time-turners travelled in a blue box (such as Lord Baker and Lord Jon Pertwee), and the bad guys in a red box (Jon Pertwee's Soul, the 'X' card, and their colleague Davros). Each were powerful in their own way and like myself they had addictive personalities. Memory is part of the skill of time-turning: complex multi-vicinity and multi-dimensional 'memory return'. Events manipulated in 'subtle vicinities', (like moulding 'K' Dimension Three) can affect the material plane because of alterations to an individual's perception and their subsequent reactions.

The best way to keep these forces on my side was to allow them to sample essences from my own throat. To give them their preferred 'rocket fuel'. Lord Jon took his tea black, and Lord Tom Baker took his tea as I did with milk and two sugars, so he was easy to please... but then there were the bad time-turners in the red TARDIS - powered by nicotine – which they could sample many times more frequently than the tea of their opposition. I was worried about the fallibility of the blue TARDIS, anxious that enemy eyes could pin it down in a subconscious group *memory return* and trap it. One Time Lord occasionally gave me help when it was really needed, who went under the name Simon Sexton but I never learnt his real name.

I learned about an inter-dimensional space called The Nexus, a Time Lord's heaven: a mental 'high', a pocket of rainbow space with a drug essence. Well, if that was what they wanted 'to tickle their sonic-screwdrivers' then that was up to them... But it became my business when I heard what The Nexus was made of: our life-force, human Phase-water stolen or purchased after an apocalypse. I tore The Nexus up on a giant *brick-through* and then made arrangements for the vicinity to be made of the essence of black tea instead. Perhaps it worked. I don't know. During a coffee break one afternoon in Walthamstow, Lord Jon advised me to make black tea in a special way. He said I would like it. After careful pouring and measuring of the drink I could distinctly smell the scent of mushrooms in the steam rising from the cup. This is the way, so I thought, to mix a true Time Lord's true tea and I drank some. A few minutes later I was getting high, a funny feeling, a skiddy rib-tickler to the brain!

After a terrible life and a good fight I believed I would inherit a place on the universal unit. Then I learned I might have a place on the Milky Way galactic plate instead – in a castle like Camelot! I had a huge fundament to use there, seated in the environs of *The Circle of Fire.* It was big enough to walk around within on the galactic: a gargantuan body that was slowly growing. There was a framework like scaffolding around its hairless head, and you know what? Drug-riddled Lower Starion *feelies* were growing the magic fungus on top of its bald pate! Climbing around the scaffold, harvesting and trading psychedelic mushrooms for credits, and that's what they'd spiked my tea with that afternoon. It was typically incorrigible!

The drugs trade was in part financing experimental Quiddity environments. It was buying feathery material from the

Micronda, Barvor bird spirits, which were being sown into spheres

that contained small hamlets of traditional English cottages. The engineers didn't know how to create realistic sky so I invented a revolving cloud projector fixed on the apex of a roof. At night a black sheath rose to cover it, which was full of holes, to project stars. My other idea was to create a recreational area - with houses and skiing and Quiddi-earth trees and grass - on the moon! It would be sealed in an electrical field atmosphere, called a 'holding cell', and it would be a place where everyone could take the shape of birds and fly in the freedom of dark skies: the Moon Bird-World!

Clive Bactu verified a bird-morphing rapture that I thought may become fashionable, catch on as a 'craze', but the simulation engineers didn't allow it. Bactu was making fix-machines also and likely a lot of credits. Harvey Keitel's *feelie*, known as 'Doctor Goo-a-Goo', was an inventor on the Lower Starion Planes and he also made a lot of money. He was a dubious father figure of mine, invented things like Quiddiere stereo players and was one of the richest souls up there. Boo ran with the ladies and seemed to have a *feelie stick* in his mouth most of the time. I discovered that Dr. Goo-a-goo had been married to a nicotine-insane deyaform called Orla Shae. They had been my parents, once, when they had killed me as an infant. The situation was getting so out of control that I did one thing for myself, and one for the plains. For myself I made an oath about the number of cigarettes that I would partake in, later in life, and for the Lower Planes I took money out of the equation: I cancelled Starion credits.

Before the law took I heard of a much more serious commodity, a Bark contract to buy a weapon being stock-piled in Gehenna: *nescrose* gas bombs to burn and poison the Alpha Perfume Ladies. I uncovered this plot when I was down there. I ripped the tail off 'Jethro', (The Thrall's #2), and even attacked The Thrall 'himself' while I was smashing up the factory floor and destroying the *nescrose*. His own shape was more defined than when I had first seen it. Instead of the appearances of a fleshy pile, or an evil blackness, or a heap of rats (the other configurations it had taken) it looked to me then like a woman and a man's body welded together. And I heard how this had happened. The story goes that long ago a married couple had been rewarded for good deeds with positions as Lord and Lady of a galactic plate and they fell asleep. Later it was uncovered that they were in fact an ancient Barker's mother and father, and were ordered off the galactic... but they had *'fatwa'd* – which in this definition means their essences had mixed together during sleep and then sank into the Asgaroth. After extraction with vacuum machines they were thrown into Gehenna as a couple welded together

which became The Thrall. Degenerating when taking drugs, it became a wobbling pile offering prophesies for a high as is written of it in '*The Nightbreed Chronicles*'. The male half was dominant. When I attacked I tried to burn his *remriece* bed and cut him with a knife. I destroyed the *nescrose* but I had also made a terrible adversary.

Bereft of their weapon Planet Bark #5 nevertheless still bayed for Alpha blood. The lady *Muandu,* Asgaroth of Centauri, declared the need for planetary aid. That day I was entertaining the possibility of a new imagination-drive made of the 'The Art Garfunkle' crystal and this energised me. So I took the position of Alpha's *Defender* because they had helped me in the past. These races were so advanced they already had one foot in the next world anyway and their space craft were inter-dimensional... since my projected-self could cross vicinities and touch them I could fight, so I went to Alpha Centauri and fought the Barks on a magnified *brick-through* from a domineering height above the planet's surface.

Fighters called 'skimmers' dropped into the pink atmosphere and attacked some out-lying villages. I snatched them out of the air and crushed them. I took on battleships in *vicinity-*

zero with imaging by Lord Jon. In the engine rooms were the ship's 'ion drives': large fluorescing tubes that I withdrew, rotated, and slid back into place, which had the affect of a self-destruct mechanism. It destroyed them within seconds. If necessary I sometimes also crashed a path diagonally up through the decks to smash a ship's main computers but the fleet wasn't defeated yet.

Bark bombers were approaching, carrying cargos of bio-hazard insects called 'gore-bees'
that terrified the Perfume Ladies. These could inflict terrible welts upon an Alpha's sensitive blue/grey skin, and sometimes death. After vicinity crossing and boarding the bombers, I encouraged the bees to attack the crew with a 'mental twinge' in the environment. Somehow they breached the flight decks. Towards the climax of the conflict I invented a hand rapture that induced the gore-bees to function in reverse. Great swarms of them flew upwards against their original program and mindlessly left the planet's atmosphere. None remained. Standing back from Centauri I then saw Barker, himself, on his own *brick-through*. He lowered a top hat to cover the planet then lifted it to reveal an infestation of Dimension Three gore-bees. Yet my hand-rapture seemed infallible and between us Muandu and I vented them all. Barker withdrew.

With our own Asgaroth now under threat I finished by grasping and crunching up the remainder of almost the entire Bark Battle Fleet in my hands. I accidentally swept up some Alpha ships but brought them back, on one of my first, and last, memory-returns! There was a ceremony, later, in a hall meshed with my bedroom. I stood in front of the President of Alpha Centauri (some agitator visualized a gun but it was a hic-cup) before a crowd of her people. For my part in winning the battle the President awarded me with a Medal Of Honour that she placed around my neck. There was applause... then I retired back to my room feeling kind of proud. It was around this time that an Alpha visited me and recorded the scent of my after-shave, *Cool Water* by

Davidoff, to synthesise and use as perfume in their atmosphere!

A few days before I was discharged from Walthamstow I split up with the princess. To me a major part of such a relationship was in the joy of writing but the palace of her father the King was an almost impossible address to post letters to. And there was another kind of long distance: that of the world of difference between our social classes. I shaved off my goatee but there was one last adventure to be had: a possible revolution was taking place outside the Hungarian Palace. The Lammarkristen's asked me what could be done and I didn't have to think about it for long: I suggested they give the people some money. It was arranged, and cash was handed out through the gates. The family were slightly dispersed: the restless mob dispersed. I split up with the Princess but I had left her, and her family, safe.

There was fighting between Cusper planes over equipment that could control levels of 'grip' over parts of my body, skirmishes won and lost, victories and defeats day to day. I had enjoyed the recovery phase of my hospitalisations in Kent and I was hoping that when I was declared 'better' I might be moved into an open ward in Walthamstow and enjoy similar carefree days. But I was discharged, to return to Colchester. In mid-May I packed the things I had left and two nurses drove me to The Lakes. That hospital 'set' at Abbeydale, with its staff mostly racist (against whites), its prison rules, its poor food and its theft, was over. My dad and I made an insurance claim against the hospital and we won! I had been a good Defender, but I was excited to be back in my hometown. I had to share a bedroom initially but the comparative freedom was another world.

There was a lot of scope for self-government in the new 'set'. Simple things like feeding the ducks that visited the back patio in the mornings, being able to make hot drinks or smoke whenever wished, visiting the shop, socializing with friends old and new, using the Art room, sitting up all night talking with *the real* people... or being able to go outside. Just sit in the garden at twilight and listen to a familiar black bird singing until he tucked his beak under his feathers. Peter told me he was God, and that I was his son. I was happy.

I used the Occupational Therapy Room a lot, which became a busy art room. Sometimes the Night Staff allowed me to paint after midnight. I began applying a newly discovered medium, water based oil colours, working my fingertips into yellow and green shades of raw paint that I called 'alien sunsets'. I also painted some traditional landscapes. When starting out a great compliment is to actually sell your work. 'Recognition' that you can do it well since aesthetes
don't usually lay out their hard-earned cash for crap. Some people might argue with that! During May I sold every 'vortex' picture I had painted the summer before, in three lots of three, with a free 'alien sunset' (sometimes carried away when it was still wet) – at £90 a throw. It felt really good!

I also discovered that I could produce autonomous 'pineals', something else that for many would feel 'really good' also – little orange balls that could transfer nicotine to themselves and radiate it. If I bent my right hand upwards, like Spiderman, they popped out from a 'ticker-tape', ejected out of my wrist one at a time. I started distributing them to encourage friendships, I actually rolled fifty of them 'down the hill' to Gehenna. They went through the gates and The Thrall allowed a few of his minions to have one or two each. For itself it made a whole suit of them and regularly wallowed in the sensation. Peter had been 'a two packs per day man' while alive. He wanted pineals for Himself so I gave Him dozens. He stuck them into His *feelie* and soon wanted more, which was demeaning...

I could understand The Thrall and his lieutenant acting this way because as demons they couldn't be expected to behave decently but Peter was supposed to be God and was waddling about with enough pineals to light a Christmas tree. I felt his dribbling demands were a disgrace, and that he had lied about his Deity. That was the worst of it. I tried to caste him into Gehenna but he bounced back venomously and continued insisting he was God. He demanded I smoke more and more. A second attempt, and then up he came again spitting offensive swear words. And so, because it seemed that nothing (and no one) could contain him, I finally caste him into Tarterous.

Some of Peter's friends had the *feelies* of gorillas: Men that in life had worn beards. They lived in 'freys' in the outer skin of *vicinity zero*. They might have asked where Peter had gone and I doubt I lied about it but I don't think I heard from him again. He may have joined one of the freys. That would have been a happier ending. The 'pineal' arrangements faded; the ticker tape probably exhausted. An argument ensued about why I should have only one natural pineal gland, like a gorilla, when every other human being on the Earth has two. Such is the power of *pushed sub-thought*. The fact is people *do* only have one!

One of the 'frey' gorillas was Zaphod Beeblebrox, of *The Hitch Hiker's Guide*. It was a book that I believed recounted a lot of historical facts. The author Douglas Adams had somehow come across true stories and factual myth about what has been called 'the old space-driving days'. The spore-assaulting robot galactic of Slarti Bartfast, another of his characters, was so old it was in fact a small Asgaroth containing just two or three shrivelled dusty worlds. Slarti was keen to catch up on old times with his friend, Zaphod. Zaphod told him that he had taken on a gorilla's *feelie* after he had died to escape from the Police! It may have been an ideal way to end this particularly tactile simulation. I don't think Slarti spore-assaulted me again.

I came across an interesting 'frey' of space gorillas from ancient Greece. They visited me on rare occasions and made me laugh. While the rest of us had been banging rocks together, with human sacrifice the height of sophistication, these guys had been theologians and artists and great philosophers. Their names had essences like: 'Bargle', 'Aristotle', 'Muttoclese,' 'Grunticular', and they basically... didn't do anything. They just sat around all day smoking feelie-sticks, lying around their fix machines getting stoned and cracking jokes and sleeping.

Enough Quiddity spirit had been returned to my spine to hold *vicinities* of my own. I sometimes held the lucid-dream destination 'Everlie', the blue skies under which telepaths could continue working or socializing while they were asleep. I also held Unit Two, a planet home to the old Richard & Charlie souls. Zaphod took a house there because he wanted a change of scene. Although the #108 soul Adrian Starliter sometimes caused trouble, it was generally a peaceable place to live.

My flat had all the things in it a bachelor needs. It was beginning to 'call' to me. I felt it was home so I couldn't have learnt much from my suffering. Things would get worse before I would accept being medicated and apply for sheltered housing. Much worse. In the meantime staying in The Lakes wasn't so bad. I was never happy for long, but tea or coffee flowed as continuously as one desired (unfortunately the bladder-locks were like granite) and some of the meal choices were pleasant. One cigarette to the next, however blocked in their own way, did keep me going. But there was one aspect missing: the prized fundamental of a woman to love me, and to understand me. I was looking for a new relationship – and she could only be a telepath.

It is a part of human nature that everybody is addicted to something. Most habits will assist you in life but obviously many can ruin it. The more harmful the substance the more unsociable it gets, and the more acceptable the habit the less it is assessed or even recognised as being an addiction. The choice of "relief core" lies within the person's unique moral boundaries. It is the common thread running through my adventures, yet when applied to heavenly bodies it is more 'cut and dried'. A relief core is an essential foundation for these. A sane old Deyaform traditionally likes coffee as a Time Lord loves tea, yet during simulation in 1998 these spirits were often depicted as being irritating and drug crazed. Even amenable compounds like salt didn't escape the vave-sim designers.

Mint-addicted feelies echoed the enemy diatribe to "teach me not to smoke" and adopted an influence over the blood-locks that made me want to smoke more. Losing a Cusper plane "Smoking Warranty" (at least twice) reinforced the placement of inter-dimensional blocks in my lungs, arteries, and heart valves. One evening I smoked seven red Marlboro, angrily lit up one after the next, to make my point, but all I felt was a brain-taste so powerful it was nauseating. Mint was not locked out, however. And I was curious. In the hospital shop I found myself reaching out for a tube of extra strong mints that I took back to the ward. I was told to call them 'tablets'. I ate one and had to admit that the affect on my blood was noticeable, and felt good, but I made no oath. The mint people said the only stuff they got was when I brushed my teeth because they had fix machines as well – when I ate a mint the 'tablets' fell out and went eagerly into their mouths. People can die from eating too many mints, and this is a typical hypocrisy: need, fix, and affect. Same old story.

One of the first singer/songwriters to have an influence on my early learning curve was Mathew Johnson of *The The*. I felt close to him and one day I discovered his feelie 'pickled' in a white circle like a giant Polo mint made of pure salt. He had been trapped in it by forces that believed if they didn't eat souls, there wouldn't be anything for them to eat at all. I rescued his feelie. I suppose my initial reaction would have been to destroy these monsters... but their environment seemed out of range of my *brick-through*-self. So I parlayed. I offered them share my lunches and dinners - with a little extra salt, and I called them 'Salty Dogs'. They ate hot food with me on a scu-line and as answers go, this was a happy one. They faded.

My psychosis evolved new challenges. Keeping the demons out of trouble, and entertained, I created the Gehennan Cinema where they could sit and watch my adventuring on a screen from the 'first person' perspective. The place seemed to be more like a social club than ever!

When my skull wasn't being threatened, when forces like the Mint People were gone, I often bowed to the Cusper Regiment. I had a 'box' shape and three 'bars' between my eyebrows – an Air-Gate sergeant – and I saluted them using my reflection. I also socialized with other patients, a strong suit of that 'set', felt a sense of holiday in the microcosm of that 'life'. I carried out bowls of hot food into the garden. After the heat of an early summer day cold showers were refreshing, clean clothes felt nice, and my Davidoff smelt pleasant and ready for anything, a scent I wore with an indefinable sense of pride. Sometimes water was also a defensive measure.

I leant over the sink and vented spore through my teeth, twisting the tap from hot to cold. Lord Jon raptured the stuff that had phase-water into spore rabbits. In showers I imagined the water washing 'through' my body, sluicing through my head as though it wasn't there to rid myself of Dimension Two. The stuff is heavy inside a telepath's body that often goes unrecognised because it's been there so many years. It may induce dark thoughts and it can creep insidiously through the bones of a skeleton. The word raptures I discovered "Tiromasu" and "Bernard Manning" (!)

opened my jaws while my head rid itself of the evil porridge, pouring it out in an invisible gush. My head did feel lighter and once its texture and weight had had the essence of an abandoned nest. I stepped out of the shower with that feeling of a thick, papery, head - rid of Dimension Two - and it should have been a good thing yet I was worried enough about my skull already. It had just felt too *different* to be good. My bladder was sometimes so blocked by scu I had to piss in a sink.

With a venomous delivery masquerading as my own anger and coming up my own sub-thought column I sometimes lost control. The anger was introspective and never aimed at anybody in vicinity one. My language was atrocious. I used to spit and shout and smack my forehead against doors and mirrors. This behaviour was due to what became known as a "Don't care / Fuck off, power-brain." but it never lasted for long and I was usually apologetic. But I was introduced to a Jewish French woman named Touleal De Santa Maria and figured that life wasn't all bad.

We talked and I learned she was pretty. Her enemy was Morton Harket, lead singer of the pop group *AH HA*. I've enjoyed their music and by all accounts Morton is a Christian man who doesn't drink much more than water. He wouldn't say "boo to a goose." His being an enemy of Touleal, and a racist, is unlikely yet I believed it as I accepted all of the crap and rubbish I heard. In this example more so because I heard it from Touleal. On a live *interlace*-line one night I saved her, and possibly her father, from being blown up in a car bomb. She bestowed her Paris address marking the beginning of our relationship, the moment for me to start to write. I used to listen to my headphones while composing letters to her and she used to read them from "over my shoulder". I drew funny doodles and attempted a few words of French. She taught me the phrase "Je t'aime". These words should have meant much more to me than just some foreign expression but sadly the enemy made the pronunciation sound beyond my reach and a bit silly. But it means: "I love you".

On 12th June, I was discharged from The Lakes and moved a step closer to returning to my own flat. Before the final gate could be opened the 'quacks' agreed that I needed to practise 'life-skills' so I was transferred to the Colchester Assessment Centre, a rather beautiful place beside a church up on the Ipswich Road. I was given the keys and unpacked my things then went to socialize. The place was still classified as a hospital and I was still on a Section Three. The staff were on duty 24 / 7 and the decor was lavish, the furniture squashy and comfortable, the seats like old slippers. Looking back in comparison the chairs in The Lakes had been like skeletal man-traps! There was all the amenities, of course; stereo, television; a bathroom (with a separate 'power' shower downstairs) a conservatory and a spacious shared kitchen. We would be responsible for cooking our own meals.

At the back of the house was a corridor formed of overhanging grape vine, in a pretty garden. I spent time there. There was a picnic table and I sometimes sat there and chatted with my 'voices' but I needed to reach my spiritual self and move properly into those sun-blessed days. The light burned through the cobwebs and unclogged my reality. Although I was still being spore-assaulted; though my illness still grasped like it was preventing my exit from a mad carnival ride, I also sensed the proximity of spiritual peace.

I have experienced flashes of interest in 'New Age' practices on and off for years. Yoga, candle and incense burning, crystals, healing, massage, and dreams; I wanted to learn more so I re-visited a shop in Colchester called *IGIGI*, an organised yet cluttered place like the paint left on an artist's palate chaotically attaining the appearance of being art itself. I looked along the shelves keenly. Standing in a swirl of incense and relaxing music I found a book called: "A guide to modern Celtic Shamanism" by D.J Conway. Was this a master's guidance? I bought it and began to read it as dedicatedly as though I was the author's student myself.

I believed seeing 'auras', such as in the example of Kirlian photography, had been another faculty taken from me by Barker when I was little. Sitting in the garden, one day, I enjoyed seeing them for maybe the first and last time. Healthy grass had an aura of pale white. Dead tree branches (in spite of thinking it was a nonsense invention that I so wanted to believe) appeared to be glowing red. With my legs tucked under me in an essence of comfortable prayer I watched a bee land on the flower of a lavender bush. The creature had been red and when its pouches were plump it turned blue and flew away!

I bought more water-based oil colours and a new easel to use in the conservatory. It seemed other people rarely used the room. After taking the precautions of laying a plastic sheet and some throws on the carpet, I started painting again. Grand Master Gaugin had visited me in The Lakes earlier that year up from Gehenna to crazily criticise the work in progress. During the credit binge in February I had bought a book of his called "Gaugin, By Himself". It's currently on a shelf in my mother's studio. I never read it.

I have an ability to paint skies from imagination and the *feelie* of Artist Damien Hirst occasionally attended me. It was agreed that my realist paintings particularly 'had good feeling in them' and others seemed to like them. The fire-related pictures were a botch up of dirty paint that showed no richness of raw colour or contrast, but I did not give up. Of the finer paintings the 'good feeling' Mr Hurst spoke about resulted in the good feeling of self-esteem. Some people say that pride is a sin but in the example of a person who has lost all their confidence through mental illness, I say that pride is good. Much of what they have lost can return - through love - beginning with the love of themselves. The final stage of their recovery is to be in a relationship with a person who loves them back as much.

I learned Touleal's true surname was Da Ponsa, and I wanted her to be my woman. She felt strongly towards me and was shortly to become separated from her long time loved one Gerard Depardieu. As a French citizen she was part of a quintessentially romantic nation. She was thirty and beautiful, with long, dark, curly, hair, and our song was called "Truly, Madly, Deeply" by *Savage Garden.* Looking at me in mirrors on a full scu-lock, we often kissed each other in the glass. Touleal often accompanied me when I went gambling and I learnt she enjoyed quality soup and tea from a silver pot.

Money was a problem. For a while in The Lakes when I had expected a wire transfer of currency into my account, I had regularly rang my telephone banking service but the balance never changed; it was mostly overdrawn! At least twice there had been a vave-sim delivery of cash, perhaps from the BBC, on its way to the hospital - and once to Thornfield Court where I had brought presents and lots of beer before being taken away by the police. It never arrived, it never even existed. Since the Assessment Centre was still classified a hospital I could only get the lowest of DSS benefits. I was ripe for the possibility of another delivery, and this time I was really going to fight for it.

The mirage of riches began with a message from London. A telepath *Fremen* called Tom, one of my black body-guards (beneath actor Morgan Freeman, a true friend of mine in past 'policies') was on his way from the capitol carrying a fat present of £50,000 in a dribble-proof bag! He was on his way south-east and I had a cup of black tea to encourage the Time Lord's assistance who passed on some of the essence to Tom's scu to encourage his enthusiasm. The enemy went to work. Coming down the A11 Tom was assailed with threats, illusions, and *pushed-sub* thoughts. I had more tea to alleviate his doubts, but when he was on the A12 the situation became more real...and more dangerous.

Two telepath police officers drove up behind Tom's car. They knew about the money and pulled him over with a brief hoot of their siren and a flash of strobes. They 'said' nothing. On the hard shoulder they walked up beside the driver's side of Tom's car and asked him to get out. Then they hit him and kicked him repeatedly and there was nothing I could do. They beat him up then drove off with the money, leaving him for dead.

The danger of renegade telepathic policemen working my home town, and the latency of the harm they were capable of, was an issue that never came up. In that reality Tom had hidden behind his *own* vave-simulation. He had creatively visualised the whole crisis as a cover to thieve the bag! He was actually on his way back to London but the BBC got the last laugh because they had rendered the bills useless. They had marked the money because they had never trusted Tom in the first place. As for me I had been marked from the beginning myself, also: to remain poor and disappointed!

CHAPTER TWENTY FIVE – <u>JULY, 1998</u>

A schizophrenic suffering 'voices' is never alone, but everyone has their ups and downs
and life goes on. If I hadn't been allowed to paint or go to town, *first vicinity* life at the Assessment Centre would have been lacklustre. There were only menial jobs to alleviate the boredom. Our kitchen was large, but it was lifeless. That holiday sensation I felt in The Lakes I also felt occasionally at the Assessment Centre but the 'life skills' thing there was like a sabbatical, with illusory decisions. I was due to contest my Section Three before a tribunal and soon I would go back to Thornfield Court. I would return there like a racing pigeon that knows no other destination and make a nest, again, up against the grind stone.

One of the things I used to do before moving to the Center was watch the birds on the pond outside the General Hospital. I liked to see the unpredictability of the ducks and coots, and the way they rippled the water behind their paddles had been slightly mesmerising. Focussing the lenses of a pair of compact binoculars on the birds until they appeared sharp and huge, the sunlight scattered into a billion bright shapes. Alfred Hitchcock's feelie gave me some 'film-making' awards but the demons and nutters watching the Gehenan Cinema could only take so much of my feathered friends. The first person view of my life had become boring to them. It was dismantled.

Between Gehenna and a vicinity-one mesh near the Cuspers yawned an abyss beneath a broken bridge that had no middle span. I imagined armaments for the Cuspers to take pot-shots at them out of Dimension Three. In a shower I made rocket launchers that my 'K' Reacher automatically outfitted with buttons and switches of exceptional detail. The Cuspers fired them gleefully at the Gehennan Gates! The demons tried a new method of crossing the divide. The Thrall's troops shrunk themselves on brick-downs and crawled up a pipeline probably made of *The Art*. This pipe was attached to the big toe of my right foot, the beach-head of their assault, and I spent many moments trying to snap off this *'Toe Loop'*, unplug it, or bust it in half. The image seemed reinforced, maybe adhered by 'memory return'.

An attentive feelie with a beard and spectacles introduced himself as Boyer. If I had felt a clash of personalities I would have had to suppress it because he was God. And He decided to initiate the Judgment Day - right from the garden of The Assessment Center! A vortex opened up and sucked down the rejected, who knew they had been convicted since each started to hallucinate a piece of grotty tissue. I don't remember who 'won' between the sheep and goats. If Touleal had been hard judged by I would have a memory of it, and I might have been worried about going down that plug-hole myself. I was 50% sure that Boyer was not The One True God, that he was an assistant, but as far as 'Judgement Days' go the remarkableness of it was to fade. Within a week I was busy doing other things with my mind-life.

If *"Truly, Madly, Deeply"* was playing when there was no one else in the lounge I would dance with Touleal. See myself in 'black tie': a white shirt and jacket with a bow, and we would move to the music together beneath an imagined spotlight. My old soul Boo had had his girlfriends also, on the Starion planes, many of them. He had been with too many of the other *feelie's* women and his promiscuity had landed him in trouble. He had also smoked a lot and most likely flaunted the laws of this issue. Standing at a bus stop a decision regarding Boo was forced onto me, which was simple even if I didn't want to know. Another kind of vortex was yawning open under Boo, black and swirling in the cold concrete beside the bus shelter. And I answered the question: *I do not want him nullified.* That would have been an extremity of injustice so I put him into Gehenna instead. Later I would understand just how horrendous that place really was. By then it would be too late.

Sometimes I encouraged my lovely Touleal to 'go do something else' while I was gambling. When she did accompany me I told her that slot machines were fun. She liked a TV monitor game in which you had to line up three cars to win a feature. She called it 'Magic Cars' but in my search for a higher paying feature fun was made into a lie as even the funny little Magic Cars could be lost, and I was embarrassing myself. I felt dirty inside, guilt in maybe the worst place someone can feel the muck. But I couldn't walk away from a machine if it 'owed me' and I still had money left to play it with. Whether Deep Set Program #16 was real or not is a moot point: I was an addict, had been for years. And it was not 'fun'. As the money disappeared I felt like I was making a mockery of Touleal's naivety. I didn't know it then but an oath would be required in order to claw my return to spirituality.

In my 'spirit quest' during the sunny days at The Center I was studying D.J Conway's *"Guide to Modern Celtic Shamanism"*. I learnt about Shamanic tools; a meditation rug, a rhythm maker such as a drum or 'bell stick', and the 'crane bag' to put things in. My reach was that the author was a woman - probably called Denise, Joanna... but in simulation I was introduced to a male author: David, Jonas, a father of mine from long ago and a dubious character. In what was probably an enemy initiative to ruin my 'quest' he confessed that he had been using his influence as a guru for sex and money. I told him to clean up his act, to forgive himself and recover the innocent approach with which he had set out. He faded.

Sitting in the smoking lounge one afternoon my Reacher started talking. I was shocked! She told me her name was Olive and that she had been operating this device within me for many years - apparently without articulating a word. Later she was 'Sarah' but that wasn't the problem. The problem was that 'Sarah' became destructive on seeing this raptured spanner materializing in front of her. When it appeared she had an uncontrollable urge to just pick it up and smash up the Reacher. I went on a campaign for an automated version. Similar happened to the White Art, my power-Art assistance for painting and writing. It was a soft material with creative abilities that had been part of the reward-base I had constructed in The Lakes. It started talking to me as well. Initially it was the native American god 'Quexicotle' because it had heard chanting while I had been asleep, and later the enemy made it into a paste. They started to wipe onto the inside of my skull to block porous venting, which heightened my fear of spore. Sarah left my Reacher alone. I have to assume that the enemy only allowed a genuine Reach when it suited them – and falsified many of my own.

The rapturer that had attacked me at the end of 1997, the 'X-Card' Paul Nicolau, had actually been the feelie of a BBC Radio One D.J: *Jo Whiley!* Of all the forces, many were in dread of her. With a 'pick-set' she could truss you up and present you like a basted turkey in a matter of seconds. She travelled in the blue TARDIS. They called her Lady Jo, and she and Touleal and I started talking together. I asked her if she would teach me some hand-raptures and she said it was OK. I had been worried that Jo may suddenly revert into a black cataclysm but we became friends. *Make a fist with your dominant hand and imagine it is 'vicinity-meshed' with your left-hand heart. Gradually open your fist, pushing out any impediments, until your hand is fully extended; then the "heart cleaner" rapture is completed.* I was eager to learn others but the enemy didn't allow it. Lady Jo wanted to be a retainer of Touleal and myself when we became *feelies* ourselves!

The manipulation of time wasn't only a faculty of Time Lords. The enemy could construct rooms that were encased a line of slow hours called an *Out Of Time Hole*. For many weeks there had been a feelie (or disconnected scu) of director David Cronenberg delving into my inner vicinities. He sometimes studied in such a hole. The by-word then had been *'genetics'*. Cronenberg, inventor of the *interlace* communication system was within me, searching dusty corners, behind doors; under crystals plucked from my *phase water* reservoir, and in the nooks and crannies of redundant battle platforms, looking for the connection between DNA and the future. He wanted the secret of Lady Nature's designs. Every time he thought he had found a new 'socket' with access to my future he took out his printer. Yet everything he ever printed out had been the destiny-line of Barker???

Shortly before I left The Lakes I told Cronenberg that what he was seeking was connected to a bath towel and I pretended I had let slip a great secret. I had lied; I did that sometimes when teasing the enemy. So off he went to an out-of-time-hole where he studied bath towels for the equivalent of seventeen weeks! He considered towel construction and the weave and texture of materials, and other details - but learned nothing - except that in this example DNA could also mean Deliberately Not Applicable! But he didn't stop. In August he would arrive at an answer. I was occupied but forgetting him had not meant that he hadn't always been there in me, and always searching.

In a typical vave-sim I was riding a bus back to the Assessment Centre and did some accidental alchemy. I merged some 'silver' with rapture crystal – probably *Mythril* from the Sheild Dome with Art Garfunkle – and made a new metal. This could talk also! The *feelie* of Thorin Oakenshield, the Master Metalurgist who had lived long ago on a planet called Middle Earth (told about in *The Hobbit by JRR Tolkien*) told me that he loved the new metal. It wasn't that it had power, which it undeniably had, it was that it was as beautiful and as malleable as gold. Thorin called it 'gildenstone'. Logical progression based on my having discovered a new source of untapped power was cancelled by the vave-sim designers. It faded within a day.

Tea bags not far away I learned enthusiastically that some genuine cash money was on its way. Mr Leonard Nimoy and

Mr William Shatner (from the original *Star Trek* series) were on an aeroplane and wanted to assist me – with about seventy grand! Unlike a wire-transfer I could make a difference in vicinity when using a live interlace. They landed at about half 10.30pm, and in fear of currency smuggling Mr Shatner had hidden several packets of cash in his sweater before he passed through the Nothing To Declare channel in customs! Irrespective of my wishes, the two celebrities were brave but they couldn't foresee how it would end. I drank black tea to nudge and encouraged their *scu's*. They came onto the A12 and most locals seeing their Limousine would have thought it exotic; to many the sight would have seemed as bizarre as a Star Ship itself! But it was real. On the outskirts of town they got lost in an area called Lexden. I had to 'get my head together' because my directions involved crossing part of central Colchester. *'Lexden'* became an expression that just meant 'lost' generally... somehow I got them back on the right road.

I offered them a few of my paintings. In spite of their increasing nervousness they said they liked that idea, so I went into the conservatory and signed some, maybe with personal messages. The Limo was coming up the Ipswich Road; they were getting closer and closer.

In spite of my battle for their well-being I was told they didn't want to meet me face to face anymore. I slipped outside to look for a place to make the exchange. By the entrance to the graveyard, next door, was a wooden notice board shaped like a wishing well. I may have left my art-work there. About twenty minutes later I crept out to fetch the money. I was excited but nothing had changed. They were still probably lost in 'Lexden'. Again I got them back onto the right road and I found a new place for the swap: by the front entrance gate in a yellow plastic 'salt / grit' box that probably hadn't been opened for several months.

I left the paintings there and soon the Limo was near. I felt like I'd been fighting for this for hours and hours, but it was a huge reward, more money than I had seen in my entire life. At last it was done. I was told they had taken the paintings;

that the money was in the grit box and they were on their way back to London. I went outside. Where to my horror I found that once again nothing had changed for the second and final time. I deflated like a stock market crash. I had to accept that they were going back to London. There was no money, and there *would be no money*. So I went upstairs and I got into bed feeling like a very old man. I slept.

That month Touleal and I went to a fayre in sunny Castle Park. I put up one of my paintings as a prize in a draw by the charity MIND. We walked from stall to stall, full of games and bargains, on a 'two-in-one'. People old and young were bustling about happily and I bought two luxury candles. We had a lovely time. My tribunal was due on July 25th but my Section Three had already elapsed so the meeting wasn't required. It was called off and a few days later my return into the community got the 'rubber stamp'. I started packing with thoughts of home; the tall windows, the kitchen, the space. I was still trashing my medication but I felt ready for the responsibility of returning to Flat 12. My enemies were prepared also. I couldn't foresee the future of my conflict there but the place wasn't called 'Thornfield Court' for an empty cup: it contained slow poison and I was going to drink it.

CHAPTER TWENTY SIX – <u>AUGUST: 1998</u>

The place looked good. The carpet was stained but Dad had cleared the rooms and there was an eager promise in the space created. We had to purchase a bed and bought a double with pipes that curled at each end like white tree roots. Like most single people I felt a comfortable anticipation about the extra bed space! My King Charles Cocker Spaniel, Lotti, moved back in and I put her wicker basket in my bedroom. I used to walk her in a field down the road, her fluffy tail wagging to and fro like a feather duster. The weather was enjoyable and sometimes I carried along a bean-bag to put on the grass while I continued to study shamanism. Lotti ran around according to the whims of her little brain. One night she lay on my bed and I went to sleep holding her paw. There was much love in that little dog.

I learned the author of *A Guide to Modern Celtic Shamanism* was a woman named Duadu. She blessed me with her council, yet rarely. I had an idea on a bus for Naturals to accept telepathy. If celebrities studied *wicka* and sorcery, magical rites – if they all moulded themselves into white and black witches in vicinity one – the public would read about it and accept that their stars were witches and warlocks in the material plane – and then see them acting the *same subject* in the movies, which would link fantasy with reality. Colchester built a new police station in 1990. It looks like a fortress.

I sometimes walked my dog around a lake down the road. Wooden platforms have been constructed at the water's edge for private fishing. At one of them I 'role-played' the god of *The Feelie Ball Of Wonder*, a beautiful idea that everybody will be in a gargantuan sphere of Quiddity after a million eons have passed us into the long future. A god will stay to look after it and I believed (as it was my idea) I would be the god to do it. I lost a digital watch of quality around the same platform. On a particularly hot day I went skinny-dipping and got banned by a warden from visiting the lake again, a few days later!

During the trauma of April '97, Boo had been the feelie *of the man I had been* before I heard 'voices'. That younger man had partaken in drugs, smoked strong tobacco and partied with the best. I might have tried not to think about this, but it is the reason Boo had misbehaved. And I had put him into Gehenna where he was literally shattered. A rapturer of the Black Arts used a 'pick set' to break him down into sixteen component entities. *Worm Boo* (the right hand) and *Golden Boo* (the love-routing) are examples. The damage was to prove permanent and The Thrall became the father figure of these sad creatures.

Lady Jo continued to be a good woman, a *Rapturer-Positiva*. When she wasn't about I tried to befriend the Time Lords by calling their group 'The Gentleman's Club' but it never lasted. They often behaved like fiends and attacked me with worm creatures they referred to as *botnes*. I found this word funny but my heart box areas were infected with them. They never hurt much but they had looked bizarre. Each had a little Jon Pertwee head on them and attacks were often announced with the words: "Pew Botne *purr-bore,* to left hand heart, middle heart, and right hand heart" and sometimes the worms were set on fire. The botne's skins formed into crackling squares. I seem to remember attacking the likes of Barker the same way.

On the night of August 16th I went into the garden to sleep under the stars. It was fresh and pleasant outside. There was almost no wind and so I lit a few candles on the grass beside my sleeping bag. We told Barker his death might be funny, like being electrocuted changing a light bulb, but I don't think it was vindictive. I felt contented, and spiritual. As the old expression goes I was "feeling my ways". I hadn't felt this lovely for years and observed a tender passion from Touleal, my friends, and my heart boxes. In the flickering light of candles like sentinel fires in the darkness, I slept well.

It must obvious to you by now that I believed I was a re-incarnation of Jesus. The original joke was that there was this psychiatrist doing his rounds one day and he asked a man why he thought he was Napoleon. The patient had replied: "God told me," then the man in the next bed had said: "No I didn't!" The whole 'anti-Christ / Jesus' thing is a common psychosis. Back in 1990 I had believed it of myself as well although I had thought I was too intelligent to be mentally ill. Self-awareness of being 'The One' (out of six billion people), of being the only mental patient in history to actually be the Lord, can seem bleak and terrible. Even when I became accustomed to it I avoided looking at myself too closely. Yet, if someone tried to bullshit me, I've been know to say: "Come off it, I wasn't born in a *shed* - not this time!"

At the worst it had been about a coming apocalypse. I had been seduced by the thunder of bass and bewitching lasers. I knew the immense power of this, which Barker had called *The Art.* I had been Lord of this dance. When I became a receiver I wanted to be acceptable and accepted, as far as I could be: an artist or writer... so I do. That needs to behave properly in front of so many attending telepaths, with so many opinions, had put me on the road to improvement and many years later, that same behaviour has helped build me into the man I am today: "Not perfect, but good," as they used to say about the Blue Vortex paintings, another example of something good emerging from the enemy's critical perception.

I had lost the license to ride my motorcycle but I rode it everywhere, and when I wasn't afraid of the police or the weather I loved every minute of it! At weekends I went down to my parents where I spent time outside. I used to walk around the grounds in the sunshine. I looked at the fully dressed trees, and the sweet flowers, and I called it 'garden therapy'. I hugged a tree with coppery leaves and I felt a soul in it of a little old man busily writing. I found a Lord in a fir tree, and when I hugged the tree beside him I found his wife, a great Lady. When I held the thin trunk of a sapling I felt a lonely baby crying. I went indoors when it started raining and came out again when it had stopped. The garden was wet and I returned to the sapling. The infant was happy now, quietly suckling water as though milk from the teat!

I bought a CD single, "Iris", by Australian band called *'The Goo-goo Dolls'* that was beautiful and haunting, like a comfortable dark place. But the band was horrible. They put dribbling shrieking dolls into my loved one's shallow sleep. I prayed sometimes to dream of her but don't remember if I did more than twice. My dreams were being invaded: Adrian Starliter was disguising himself to have sex with Touleal, and the Old Richard and Charlie souls in Unit Two were *solidifying* my dreams *and eating them!* Others complained that Starliter had been raping their women also and I almost dumped the entire planet down the toilet. But I didn't flush it: the threat had been made. I had little trouble with them after that. Anyway, most of the time I couldn't even piss properly without loosening it in showers.

I had no sedatives and used to wake up feeling more tired than I when I went to sleep. Every afternoon I got up feeling worn out because the sleep-healing chemical I unconsciously made was being stolen. Lower Starion feelies were snorting the powder to wake up. The Gehennans were using it to grout tiles in what they called The Waking Wall. If I managed to rise and take a cold shower as soon as I woke up I could recover some. I didn't mind freezing showers or baths when I was hot and sweaty - but having one immediately after getting out of bed (feeling as sluggish as that) had been grim. That's probably why the enemy encouraged the arrangement.

I didn't only ride round to my parents on weekends. During 'garden therapy' I spoke to telepath psychiatrists. One day something unexpected happened that took me into the shadow of death. Cronenberg had solved a rotating-dial and opened a vault in one of my inner vicinities. There were drawers in it like safety deposit boxes against the wall and each contained a spider with my exact genetic match of cancer of the name on the drawer. Mine was found I had believed it was over, then, to be an air-death for me: over. In spite of having been a good Defender – fighting for over seventeen months and even destroying the Helter Incendo of London - I was marked and fell to my knees with the loudest protest of "**why**!?" Then discovered the surprising truth of the matter. Cronenberg had learned weeks before that Barker's DNA signature was in my body. So my spider was taken away and rubbed into his lungs by the Fremen. Inside him was a spider that was the exact genetic match of Harlan Ellison's, and that was rubbed into his; and in Ellison's was the cancerous spider matching the DNA of Terence Stamp. So the enemy started falling like nine pins… and you know what I learned after that? My genetic match of cancer did not even exist!

My parents got back from holiday on Tuesday August 18th and I rode round that evening like a blood hound on the scent of Duty Free tobacco. After dinner I went back to Thornfield Court, probably a carton of Marlboro better off, which would free up some extra cash for gambling. I started playing the slots again. The noise of pound coins spilling into the tray, the free coffee, the buttons and the blurred spinning fruits was as entrancing as ever. The Los Angeles vicinity "Everlie" had a room added that indicated the breadth of my influence, with gaming machines of their own. Regular players let me into a secret that *Scu* could induce jackpots. They could use a wafer thin (and dubious) vicinity mesh with the material plane – but my enemy could put this in reverse.

After playing hard on games that logically 'owed me', the enemy would scramble them and ruin any chance of recovery. And again I felt that deep dirt: the clash of spirituality with obscene materialism. It may have been the first time anyone had ever actually said in plain terms that the war in these days was about: **guilt verses happiness**. Years ago I had said that "guilt is a waste if emotion"… Maybe only good people are hurt by it. And a few times the enemy said something else I couldn't grasp: that when I was *happy* they couldn't touch me. Although I was hardly ever happy in those days, I understand this now. Presently I am happy almost all the time. There is truth in what they had said.

Gambling was like going back again and again to the pipe and I needed to rein it in because I was ruining myself. I needed to shrug off the heavy stench of guilt. So I found myself looking out over the lake on a fishing platform, leaning into the hot sun for a purer moment and made an oath: When I am married I will play only an *agreed amount*, with my wife, and no more [AMMENDED TO OUR BEING ENGAGED AS FIANCES] but until then, from that 'now' moment beside the water, I said I would stop gambling. And that heavy muck fell from my shoulders. It felt good.

I had genetic engineers working for me, moulding my future with computers made of an unknown material I was familiar with the problem that given enough time they went wrong, started programming traffic accidents and assassinations and diseases. I wanted rid of them. One morning I woke up with a strange new friend, a raptured phase-water bag that was plump and talkative called *Deeply Love*. He knew the histories of many old 'triax policies'. His understanding of genetics must have exceeded even Cronenberg's. He had knowledge of the passed lives of many and it all demanded respect.

Deeply Love used to work in a vicinity manipulating genuine genetics. My loved one's wobbly phase-water bag arrived soon after that, called *Deeply Do* (from the lyrics in our song by Savage Garden) and she in her turn knew a lot about Touleal. Then two more popped up: Barker's bag was called "Deeply Hate" and Ellison's "Deeply Blood", named since its phase-water was as red as the nature of the man himself. It was interesting. They showed none of the animosity of the people they served. All the bags got along well and Deeply Love and Deeply Hate particularly showed a respect of each other that seemed almost clique. They talked and threw rapture coins back and forth. If Deeply Hate threw a double headed coin at Deeply Love it would be thrown straight back at him, as though they had known each other and days like these before...

On the night of Thursday 19th Deeply Love and God created a tool. It was designed to even the odds. After working on it for 10,000 years in an out-of-time-hole they emerged with a system that could grow on the brain called *The Nine Device*. When the neural nets achieved the maximum fixed position the system could deliver *all known raptures*. It could attack and defend without need for jargon because it used plain English. There were some initial problems with it developing 'illegal personalities' but good straight talk to it helped no end. I could feel it, on the top of my brain; and from the 20th I occasionally fought with it.

Touleal believed that I was a re-incarnation of Oscar Schindler, the saviour of many Jews in the Second World War. Others thought that I had been Martin Luther King. In my turn I believed that Touleal was the *reflection*, and the *re-incarnation*, of a horrible sister long gone. A few nights before I grew *The Nine Device* Touleal and I had enjoyed sex with Love Talkie Pearls. It had been lovely. With the seasonable warmth I rode to Friday Woods with a carton of orange juice, some sausages and two cans of beer. I walked into the trees where I found a place of grass that seemed like a green nest. I lay down my sleeping bag and most likely had Fred with me.

While I was collecting dry sticks for the fire I made a mistake. I tore a green branch from a living tree - and when I tried to light it I couldn't get a flame going. Even with dried leaves it wouldn't catch so I felt I should apologise to the spirits of the forest, for hurting the tree.
I did. The fire caught immediately into crackling flames. The enemy could not have simulated this. That night there had been a lot less conversation than I had expected, thoughts that the enemy didn't want me to talk to anyone. I wondered if the Army would come into my glade on exercise and point

blank rounds at me in their SA 80s. I fell asleep. Other than myself, the only living things in the forest that night had been nocturnal: flying with light intensifying eyes; or shuffling along in warm darkness like the way I saw sleep coming when I'm tired. I don't remember any dreams. Sleeping with that feeling of being a part of the raw earth of the forest may have been like a dream in itself.

The obscenely body-pierced demons in Barker's film *Hellraiser* existed in undesignated vicinity. Through my alphabet the word *Cenobite* can mean: "see 'E' no, *bite*", which has the essence of a withdrawal experienced beyond this world. Consequently, the Tarteran *'Pin Head'* (soul of actor Doug Bradley) never took any substances most people would consider addictive. He liked pork fat. I shared it with him to curry favours, pork curry obviously. My enemies had said God was *porcine*, like the British Police are sometimes called pigs, and it goes a long way to explain why a demon would want to eat it. He took the meat on a scu-lock and later with a fix-machine. He attacked Stargore or Gehenna for me sometimes after taking his of pork chops, bacon, scratchings, luncheon meat, sausages, gammon, crackling, pork pies, sliced ham... I'll write it again – everybody has their addiction!

After all the years that had been invested in *The Nine Device,* it was sad when it went the way of all simulations and was cancelled. Meeting friends in Vagabonds Café a speck of the device was taken from my head and put into Barker's. It grew on top of his brain as it had done with mine, and at max-headroom he had identical capability. Within two days both devices were somehow reduced to nothing. Another sad occurrence was when I had to accept that I couldn't be a shaman. After the destruction of my *imager* I couldn't meditate. There was just a dim redness there and since spiritual growth in shamanism is deeply rooted in meditation I had to give up my studies and it was like the end of summer.

My castle would look like Camelot and it was being built by Barks on the Milky Way Galactic Asgaroth. After I heard that the aliens were being poorly paid and whipped to the task I halted the work. Having forgotten that I had banned Starion Credits, already, I paid for all the Barks to have a feelie stick and a cup of tea out of my own bank-roll. Whether a test of my views on slavery, or my feelings for Barks, I knew I had done well. Barker high-jacked my gigantic *fundament body* a few times to rapture it to bits or smash up the castle. The fundament had taken so long to grow and the castle so long to build I found this distressing but I felt impotent to stop him.

The castles of others were often cemented block by block into simulation. After an apocalypse the Cuspers had lived in a castle for 50,000 years, which I assumed was a 'reward' for acts of darkness. Some Alphas were building a miniature castle paid for by Harlan Ellison, a tiny platform to spore assault me on a brick-down *from within* my skull. Another castle was being built by a transient god that seemed to be designed to prevent me seeing Touleal. I smashed it up. Apparently he didn't understand sex so he was transferred to another Unit in my spine where he became god of a planet of feelie babies!

In spite of my protests to the contrary I had been called *'a feelie gone wrong'*. Attending scu and souls had thought that my washing the dishes was an evil ritual since they had magic plates, cutlery that washed themselves, and they revered water. In the kitchen, I eventually had to explain that we do our washing up manually, with our hands or a machine – and that it is perfectly natural. When they saw the container of washing-up liquid they had an epiphany, a bottle of "Fairy" with the baby scampering across the front. "We understand now," one of them said. "People live in hell." And I replied: "No. We just make the best of it."

It was good that those attending grasped this. It was another example of making friends out of enemies but their reaction was short lived. Barker came into alter memory, to wipe the event as though it had never happened. Recollections are crucial to feelies and, in the form of a record, very important to myself also. I didn't want to be haunted by annihilated achievements. For a while memory manipulation was flavour of the month – again – until, for the second time, the souls on the Lower planes started painting their memory cards to assist their recall.

Many days were front stage for the attacks of *Worm Boo,* a chip from the old Boo soul that had been broken to pieces. I had cut him in half; he drew himself together. He hated me probably only a little less than he hated himself; a worm that attacked in many ways and in any way possible. With the exception of the spore I was subjected to that everyday, the heavier forces only assaulted me when I was doing well. One afternoon Barker attacked with a particular viciousness, released a weapon called a *sporande virus.* He wasn't after me, he wanted the destruction of feelie planes and his motive may have been for me to be blamed. I don't know. But whatever the reason the virus cut a swathe along the planetary systems of distant stars and I was at a loss. Hundreds of thousands were dying. Then up popped Lord Jon Pertwee, leaping to the rescue with a *Grand Massive Time Turn* that cancelled the contagion.

He rejuvenated the feelie victims and cleansed the virus from the Time Lines. You can bet your bottom space credit I gave him a cup of tea for that one!

The general behaviour of the Time Lords was a mess. If I brewed black tea, happy moments never lasted long because of their outrageous demands, like: "if you don't drink black tea every five minutes for the rest your life we'll kill you." And I found the taste of it had piquancy like chewing a daffodil stem. A singer called Martika, who had released an album called *Martika's Kitchen*, declared her real kitchen 'open house' for the Time Lords because she wanted "to do her bit". But she couldn't cope either. If I knew the Time Lords they had probably been sucking at different drinks like dribbling maniacs, never giving the poor woman a moment's peace.

While I was in the kitchen, quenching my thirst directly from a tap, something amazing happened. I imagined an alchemy in my throat, a filter that changed *Escent One* (water) into *Quiddity!* I was advised to drink a little at bed-time, to supplement my dreams. It was considered miraculous but if

287

you are expecting something went wrong you are right. A new form of dependency was created over which I had virtually no control. Addiction was a problem already but the filtering process made *Quiddi-filtered artefacts*. Hyper-addictive feelie-sticks and drinks were created and fix-machines were coughing up different coloured pills and drug tablets for that "fix when you want" freedom. Once more I was supplying junk against my wishes.

My friend Deeply Love said that this was the worst life I had ever led. Sometimes, he dreamt me experiences from past 'polices'. I had a vision of a night long ago when I was walking with Charlie Jordan and some other DJs. We were friends. It was lovely to be with her, talking to her as I had never had the opportunity to do in this life. I noticed my head was delicate and "boat shaped" that, compared to the strength of today, we all had the fragile skulls of aliens – *we were aliens!* In another dream I was a bar tender in New York, in a gang that fought against Barker's gang. Sadly at the end of this vision I witnessed, 'again', my good friend Morgan Freeman being shot; killed alongside friends I didn't recognise but had known, people whose names have gone long ago into the twilight files of history.

As I had for Charlie the year before, I wrote regularly to Touleal and sometimes I enjoyed it. I don't remember the enemy trying to prevent it, stopping letters being sent to a real person that was actually going to read them, if you follow me? Yet I kissed Touleal sensually in mirrors and shared my crushing existence with her; a life about the extremes of love and terror. I felt Touleal's feelings for me like warmth to a man whose enemies have had him cryogenically frozen.

According to Deeply Love I had lived many lives: 1000 as fish, 2000 birds, 2000 animals and many thousands as people. Everybody has had many lives. At our current stage in evolution, he said, everybody existed in a common genetic structure perhaps extracted from Dimension Two. We were living in the same houses with the same families in the same locations, had the same friends and the same jobs. Yet Deeply Love also revealed that our planet was moving into a time that we have never had before. We were moving toward a new age of survival and self-government beyond the final year of the oldest recorded 'policy'. It cued a mystery trajectory for the Earth people to take the reigns themselves and forever overcome the horrors of the Triax policy System.

The larger part of my own war was making people happy, to make friends out of enemies. Since he hated himself so much I arranged for Worm Boo to be reformed to his liking and he accepted a hermaphrodite body with a pink ballet Tu Tu... It takes all kinds! A couple of times I rode to a nature reserve to treat those attending me to bird watching. It seemed like a long time since Sandy and I had visited the place on that sunny day. At the reserve I walked along a pontoon and into a wooden hide that overhangs the edge of the mud. I took out my binoculars and observed some gulls and wading birds. I didn't take a Thermos but if I had the Time Lords would almost certainly have interfered. They would have forced me into bringing black tea in at least a two gallon bucket!

The extreme high of a Quiddi-filtered artifact was like lying on a beach of diamonds under the stars, undeserved; so the higher powers altered that into hallucinations of toilet stuff. The tablets dropped out of the fix-machines and the addicts took them because in spite of the sewage the high was the same. In Vagabonds café I once had a few puffs of a cigarette and drank some iced Coca Cola and created a particularly 'phat' purple and blue lozenge shaped pill... which got the addicts sky-high while I was in the Gents for that truly "largin it multiple vicinity toilet experience!" As for the Time Lords, they all but disappeared. Retired into a reservoir of Quiddi-filtered drinks floating obliviously around and round in my middle heart-box. Although they most likely wanted to be left alone there I was having trouble 'letting them go' in my own mind because they had been a part of my conflict for so long. New antagonists came and they also sometimes left as friends.

Worm Boo had wound me up chronically, a tiny yet formidable enemy. His hatred of me was about jealousy, and maybe also about the hatred of his own physical identity. Yet he was happy with his transsexual body and next I demanded that he go under the name of Mr Clements. He became a friend. As I wrote in my notes: he knew who had helped him and he knew who had hurt him. The enemy de-raptured him back into his worm self, a typical frustration, but I doubt he ever attacked me again as he had already.

Life would have been easier if Deeply Love hadn't posted scenes to Touleal I would rather have kept private. Scenes of my dubious early sex life or crapping in the bath as a toddler were not required. In return Deeply Do sent images into my sleep of Touleal she would rather have kept private, herself. These phase-water bags were very real to me so I couldn't work it out. Logic dictates that if Deeply Love was real he would never have allowed the enemy to vave-simulate himself *or* Deeply Do.

As I have said before, having a nightmare can be better than experiencing no dreams at all but I've seen some real psychotic weirdoes that bolted me awake with the need to smoke. I didn't recognise that my 'life' at Flat 12 was a hellish dream in itself. I still referred to my parents' house as 'home' but I always went back to the war, to fight through a psychosis no one could believe, understand or cure. October set in, with longer periods of darkness. The weather was colder so I set up my duvet and sleeping bag beside the gas fire in the living room, and started 'going soft' again as in days of old. I watched television in the warmth, cuddled myself in soft stuff: yet alone, always alone. The night with its occasional rain was locked outside beyond the long curtains while I repaired my armour and re-charged myself. With this R&R I could recover the fractured bits and overcome the bruising of this ceaseless conflict. After revealing the true nature of Barker I had thought it was over. Yet it continued. And I had to continue with it.

The enemy had declared "a war of attrition" against me more than once. What they did to me during 1997, their pain and manipulations and false realities, they did all of that with a secret. They had the capability to kill everyone in the world with sub-drives early the following year. It was a horrible way to die. Once, when I was trying to sleep it seemed that my skull was being inflated and deflated with my breathing. An energiser had been meshed near to my sinuses. A lot of old spore was being rejuvenated and I was breathing it in, so I had to bang out Fred. I hardly ever washed the pillowcase because I liked the cool softness, and sometimes the scent, but I had been porous venting on it for so long the material was riddled with spore dust. It was typical of the enemy to cast a shadow over something so comforting to me, yet soon the cover was washed and cleaned.

The worst vave-simulations of 1998 were nearly always a mesh of spore and invention, such as facing the possibility of a virus of sub-drives. In spite of the controller's promise that they would never again kill a human being I was given a 'live-link' to a film studio in Canada, under the duress of director David Cronenberg. I was driven into believing the unimaginable chain-reaction had begun. People were actually dying of the stuff in there. To me, it was reality. After the first death the crew sat or stood, very still. They were frozen with terror. Another died. They were looking around at each other, wondering who would be next, yet once it was revealed that I had both actually *believed* it had been happening – and that I had *no idea* how to stop it – the simulation ended. The engineers had most likely learned what they needed. Long ago I had been told there was 4% more chance of an event taking place if I believed it would...

During a similar test, when I believed that Barker had died this way, there had been a particular fear that the same spore that had killed him were in my own skull also.
I was on a knife edge. Walking around the flat with this bomb on my shoulders I heard Barker was definitely gone and that the chain reaction hadn't happened. When I learned that my own spore was venting porously I exclaimed I would have a 'T' shirt printed saying: *I Love Spore Assault Vehicles...* because, for a moment there, I had been just as crazy as batshit. Breathless mania, madness within madness. The declaration that the whole thing had been simulated meant that Barker was still alive and that the war had to continue. But it meant, also, that no one had died of the spore.

The Alpha Centaurians must have had a short memory. Forgotten that I had once kissed one of their Perfume Ladies in a mirror so passionately that she had split out of herself a little baby; a new one for you there (and new to her also!) They must also have had a memory lapse about my saving their planet while I was in Walthamstow. They sold the brick-down castle and my attacks on it had no effect. The miniature platform could be flown wherever they willed it inside my skull and if I managed to damage it was brought back through a 'memory return' so ridged it seemed to be indestructible. But it did fade. I think I wrote in my notes: "a weapon used too much loses its effectiveness". The enemy probably got bored of it after it didn't kill me.

I stayed at my parents for several days that month. I wasn't given the yellow room where the pleasure of new telepathy had soured, I was given the bedroom between my parent's and my Dad's office, the 'purple room'. The bed there had my favourite duvet on it, heavy with feathers, but getting to sleep remained difficult. I was jerked out of intensiform by laser guided attacks from an Alpha space craft. Once again the Perfume Ladies displayed forgetfulness. They were firing a gun from a ship they called the *Hexacor* that made me feel like my head was about to explode just as I was drifting off to sleep. I fired back in return with a virus but I didn't want to hurt the baby. Life would have been much easier if I had just remembered, myself, that I had helped them! I used to swig a few burning mouthfuls of cognac before switching the lights out. For a while it worked.

I returned after being introduced to the Lords *above the* Time Lords, a peer group of senior time robots. When they inevitably started sampling tea from me on a 'full lock' a problem developed – not again; no, this was *worse* than usual: They ruined my own tea by processing theirs through slim wires meshed with my brain that felt like a spore delivery mechanism. The filaments absorbed tea essence while almost none of it entered my own blood stream. They felt disgusting and creepy. I think one of these robots had said that they couldn't help the presence of a little spore. I tried to snatch a quick cuppa in their absence and often memory-returned the horrid filaments quite by myself: an accident? Doubtful. I have never had much luck with the robot nations but something amusing did happen at the café. I had the idea of asking an attending robot for any hints it might have on advanced technology for the Earth people. First it said CDs... then it said DAT cassettes... (I replied that we have those already) and then it suggested *'digital vaccination'*. And when I sussed this I thought it was such a horrendous idea I started laughing!

Back at my parent's house the *Hexacor* left its orbit. I was *not* an enemy of the Alpha Centauri – that had been clarified. The battleship was on its way home but it was recalled on a worse than customary memory return. The Hexacor's entire crew had their *minds reset* also; so it seemed they had forgotten why they had left. I was lasered again but I established a remedy, which took work, but it was recognised by my enemies when they allowed the *Hexacor* to leave. October had been a tough month but there was no battle for Halloween at the end of it. A new god called Moochar was revealed. The old pretender of July '98, Boyar, was cloned in an out-of-time-hole as part of an initiative to copy my worst enemies. I hoped that the little phase-water bag I had first known, Deeply Love, could not have sent hurtful images into Touleal's dreams. Many situations were a vave-sim of psychosis, a madness within madness. The night Deeply Love had left he had detected thoughts directly confusable with mine. I had sensed fear and yet maybe a hint that this was nothing new. He had cried some emergency code numbers up to the heavens. The next morning he was gone by the time I awoke.

I attended a 'Hearing Voices Group' early on Friday evenings about ten minutes walk from the café. It was run by a friend who suffers from schizophrenia also, that has chosen to live with his 'voices'. You have read of the torture I have suffered at the hands of mine, so you won't be surprised that I cannot. I want get rid of them. I need release because there is another life for me out there.

New technology has fascinated me. I love good sound quality, like Mini Disc players traditionally encased in metal, and compact. They have a strong essence of control over something comparatively small. You can rattle them while jogging and you can record either digitally or analogue, or directly into a mike. I took my Community Care Grant down to the Sony shop and bought one with a battery charger that doubled as an edit deck! One of my first recordings was from an album called *Ambient 74:40*, music that is outlandish and beautiful. When I was compiling it I danced like a spiritually advanced alien around my parents' kitchen on a long headphone cable! Golden Boo rose from Gehenna and he danced also, and manipulated himself to enable impossible stretches. I had mixed feelings about it. I called the disc "Alien Dancing Music" and one song was so haunting I wept over it more than once. *"Let's see 'im cry without the music on,"* the enemy used to say.

Touleal was enjoying a holiday in the Seychelles with Monsieur Depardue. They walked on white beaches that I believed were on the other side of the world. Her *scu* came to me while she was sleeping. Unless the enemy kept me up late she could only dream of me. The couple did happy things like riding a pony…I would have liked to be romantic with her myself later in life. It was good that my father had planned a holiday for ourselves.

My sister Ellie and her man lived and worked in Lanzarotte, where we were going to stay for a week (most likely between the 11th and 18th of November, none of us can remember the dates exactly). I had a picture in my head of palm trees and white sand so I visited a Travel

Agents to look at the 'winter-sun' brochures. Far from my Caribbean beach dream the island is made of blasted volcanic rock that looks more like the surface of Mars. Lanzarotte was the place NASA practised manoeuvres for the moon landings, some tactless sod told me, yet hot sun was guaranteed and I felt it was a place I could escape from the fighting. Not much chance of that, obviously.

Spore was sometimes used in conjunction with bone weakening *Ratnika*. There had been a history of at least six other ways of attempting to stress the integrity of my skull. When some had been tried initially, a very few, but some, I had thought I was going to die... 'wyra' tissue... a "'Y' frame" (pushed up my soft palate hole and opened like a car wheel jack)... "tookle 'H' gates" to hyper-space a brick-down of the favourite fish creatures of the Barvor... 'swit bursters' like hand grenades that released a mass of Dimension Two... the red laser of the *Hexacor*... and, finally, new for November '98: *The Triax Loritzer*.

The Loritzer was a pellet gun wielded by the Cusper regiment, after they had meshed some battlements with the purple room. They were not 100 feet tall but man-size, after-all. A Cusper often on the trigger of this gun was the dark half of twins named Black and White Filial. The *Loritzer* fired miniscule pellets of compressed Dimension Two that I could physically *feel* hit my brain, and they detonated on my first image in sleep. Sometimes more than one pellet was lodged into my head for an extra pressure so terrible I was sometimes briefly certain that I would die. I almost jumped out of my skin several times every night!

It was vicious and due, in part, to further amnesia regarding some of Barker's actions. He had stolen Water and Air Qualm babies to make into *scu*. This alone should have been enough to make allies of the Cuspers. Yet the Filials (particularly reflected by Black Filial) had apparently both originated from a Barker soul. At least two examples of forgetfulness may have been placed for me to redress the balance. Yet because of powerful inside influences I couldn't act on them and this generated longer suffering.

My damaged religious position could create fear. I was spore assaulted while praying, attacked if I came across church music, and I had witnessed awful vave-simulations of the Lord Jesus. I had worshipped pretenders, and I no longer went to church. One evening, I walked into my room to find the god Moochar sexually molesting Touleal's *scu*. I deposed him. Far from being God he was apparently a *muathril*, which means life created through Rapture. He was an actor made with "two bones and a sinew". Once again, I sought a new deity to pray to. In early November I was introduced to a force that I recognized could be the highest power in the universe, the force of *Telepathy*. I felt it as an essence of continuous all-knowing depth yet I found it was represented by creatures that were much easier to understand. In a vicinity that was huge, and high above us, there were sea creatures like gigantic seals but they were *not Barvor*. They had no ulterior motives. They were so relaxed they seemed ponderous and slow thinking in a lovely way. The only method that these beings could keep track of me was with the supreme force of telepathy, which they represented. It might seem paradoxical to pray to those same forces to be a non-telepath but whom better?

In spite of my "kick & kiss" approach many situations went the other way. Some new friends became enemies. Soldiers raptured out of vast tracts of *vicinity zero* space that month went into the fight, nullifying antagonists. They came to be called *Nullies*. They may not have known what to do with themselves after their job was done, but it never *was* done. They stalled, in part because of an event that was all too common. I was smoking at the moment a Nully came in to destroy my blood locks. I felt myself beginning to swell with nicotine, in a hugeness that was satisfying physically yet was worrying. I wanted to get away from these new influences and back to some semblance of normality, however nasty. I had laughed in the mirror about the excellent feeling but it was juxtaposed by the likelihood of this Nully's spontaneous addiction. Nullies were a significant factor I carried with me on holiday.

On the morning around November 11th we drove to Stansted Airport. I like trains because you can relax with your feet nearer the ground and have a lovely view through the windows, yet during air flight I have felt fear and also a sense of continuous low-grade excitement in anticipation of the holiday. The last time I had flown was returning from that ill-fated trip to Ireland in 1997. On the journey to the Canary Islands I was visited by telepathy representatives, seals at 30,000 feet. They started rubbing me with brushes, saying "We're seals! We're seals!"

Brushing me to cancel my telepathy. A seal with a broom in its flippers must surely have been a bizarre sight if anyone had gotten a good look at them, but their brushing had no effect. "We're *seals*" they often clarified happily...then went away. After we landed I learned that rubbing with brushes was actually the therapy to reduce telepathy *in a Bark*!

Our apartment was cool and layered with lots of white tiling. There was a swimming pool on the back patio. I lay on a lounger in the sun trying to read a Dean Koontz novel but my concentration wasn't consistent. Sometimes I played an LCD game of pocket roulette. I came to believe that swimming was the only time I could talk to Touleal and swam an extra length each day. The Nullies came to me regularly to be hugged. In their search for identities I decided to name some: "Julie", "Nully One", "Nully 2000" and a couple of others. I didn't want to stimulate the unknown quantity of their anger, but they came to me at odd times – like while I was sitting in our hire car – and the cuddles got out of control, seemed to be playing on my kind nature. Sometimes it was physically tiring and since I didn't want my parents to see me hugging and (probably whispering) to 'myself', I had to put a stop to it.

Nights were the worst. The bladder rapture was terrible. I plodded back and forth to the bathroom believing my pissing was being exposed to all on a World Wide Inter-lace for at least an hour every night. And I was shot with the *Triax Loritzer*, sometimes as many as sixty pellets at once. This gun had ended the lives of three Old Richards, so I was told. One had leapt off a bridge; the others likely lost to suicide also. Some pellets were tagged with images that jerked me out of sleep. Psychopathic visions like a dribbling idiocy with a demon's booming voice saying: *"Physically Insane?"* accompanying the sensation that my head was going to explode. An untreatable madness clarifying the perception of my own 'sanity'? Dad had brought a bottle of Stelazine anti-psychotics with him and I even took some but in the absence of proper night sedation I sometimes drank Malibu from the neck and that didn't work particularly well either.

We visited a small beach. I saw some nice ladies tanning themselves on sand like brown sugar. I donned a mask and a pipe and flippers, and paddled out to the rocks. I wanted something to write about to Touleal and I wanted Mum to think I was having fun. I saw an aqua-lung diver on the sea bed below me and his bubbles rose like jelly fish to disappear on the surface. I hadn't been snorkelling for a long time. My breathing sounded excessively loud, my chest felt tight, and I was aware that a wave might wash over my pipe. After virtually throwing up on a mouthful of sea water I had to return to the beach. I have used a float, such as a life-preserver, for snorkelling since. Do the same thing if you have had similar trouble.

We went on a genuine submarine that had a camera on the conning tower and small live monitors to watch it dive. We went for a ride on camels that loped gracefully for a short distance into the volcanic tundra. While sitting outside a café in the marina where Ellie worked I enjoyed drinking an iced

Coca Cola and slowly eating a small omelette that I believed was simply the best little lunch I had *ever had*. Best of all was the night halfway through the week when I was rescued from the Cusper's gun. Art Garfunkle's *scu*, soul and fundament bodies discovered a radio link between the *Triax Loritzer* and its pellets; then fiddled about inventively and created a device that blocked the signal rendering the gun useless. Most likely I went to sleep smiling – and with the chance to wake up in a way most people would consider normal – that I do not remember.

The last time I gambled was on that holiday. I was on a sun lounger playing pocket roulette and decided I would play the real thing if I could scrape up a bank-roll. So on our last Friday in Lanzarotte I filched my passport and got a lift to the sea front "to do some Christmas shopping". I walked into the casino lobby with about £47 – learned the main room wouldn't open until 8pm – and played the slots in the foyer for about an hour and a half. This was the second time I had gambled since I made the oath by the lake. I believed that a divine force I called Lady Nature was allowing me to: that isn't 100% clear but I managed to line up a few BARS and ended up better off with about £107. At eight o'clock I went through onto the gaming floor, I bought the Spanish pesetas equivalent of five stacks of twenty at a table – and I lost the whole lot within 15 minutes! I met the family at the restaurant; borrowed another £20 and lost that as well, within four spins… they knew what was going on. I can report, now, that I haven't gambled, not on cards, nor a horse or a dog, nor a lottery ticket or even *one* scratch card in four and half years. After some home spun roulette on a toy wheel for loose change, the following year, I felt bad and wound up giving all the coins back. And that's it. My life was, needless to say, different. I became sensible with my income and I haven't looked back. Strange thing is that even now I sometimes dream of playing those

machines. In such a dream I remember my oath, with surprise, and occasionally I get spore assaulted. I wonder how I came to be playing again yet figure it's too late to stop.

R.E.M maybe simpler than people think. You may dream of material things but it is *not* material plane reality.

I went through the 'Nothing To Declare' channel at the airport with ten cartons of Marlboro. That saved me a lot on British prices. Before the end of the month I was back at the flat and got a 'back claim' of Disability Living Allowance cheques. I was excited, sensible, and a rich man... for about ten minutes! I went to London on the train, alone, and bought some sexy videos and watched *'Cats'*. In Colchester, I bought a big fluffy white toy that I called 'cuddle dog' and he would become a great comforter. But I was still psychotic, the holiday was over, and I was back into the fight. The seals didn't visit me with their brushes or any other rapture to silence my mind on the flight home.

'Enemy' meant whoever I was fighting at the time. If I forgot about them they would no longer be a foe, however, hells like Stargore, Gehenna and Tarterous *weren't* going to *forget me*. I found respite in a novel by James Herbert called *The Magic Cottage,* the first I had read from cover to cover in over a year and a half. A friendly Irish woman became my 'reader' although I couldn't hear the inflections of her language because of the Accent Lock. The cottage in the story is set in a forest, with friendly birds and animals, and it's a setting I would like to live in myself later in life.

In Tarterous the 'Pin Head' cenobite trapped a young actress/singer called Martine among his demons. She was given a metal piercing in her cheeks that stopped her from *even wanting* to leave. The Boo Gimps in Gehenna slept in shoe boxes tucked up using Touleal's *scu* panties as blankets. At my parents I had a disgusting problem with The Thrall licking the private parts of Touleal's *scu*, causing her woman a rash in the material plane. An enemy asked if I still fancied her sexually in spite of the sores. I don't remember if my revenge had been affective, or not, but both demons put their tongues away and shut their filthy mouths.

As if my existence wasn't hard enough already, I soon learned there was a fourth hell called Hades. Satan wanted to enter the fray but he had missed the last twenty two months of the war and he had absolutely *no idea what was going on*. I learned in his last life he had been Napoleon, and that he was lonely. Since Touleal was French I had this idea to "get the devil off my back" and asked her *scu* if she wouldn't mind going down to be his woman. She agreed, and there was peace. Hades <u>never entered</u> the conflict.

That month there were more attempts to clone my adversaries but Lord Jon reversed the process to produce forces of goodness instead. Six Boyers flew around vicinities with wings strapped to them called 'bum bags'. They wanted to make a statement: that they were *good* people now and wanted to have their names changed to Boye. The spore attacks continued everyday and someone else thought I needed a new brain so one was created for me. A cube-like block clipped inside my head and coated in a black material that was impervious to enemy X-rays. They couldn't see through it to map the neural nets and the structure of those were a secret. It wasn't the 111 Power Brain but control was adequate and it may have even allowed me a certain amount of creative freedom.

I might have coerced 'Pin Head' into releasing Martine. He had a pork 'fix machine' now and if I enjoyed slowly chewing the meat for him sometimes an entire live suckling pig would drop out! A huge mother of a pig fell out once and he built them a sty. Pin Head's monster Gorkon puzzle box used to say "legal thought" or "illegal thought" according to my sub-statements. After a week or two of particularly juicy pork Pin Head constructed the *Rose Gorkon*, my own box to defend my cubular power brain. The vave-sim engineers may have thought I had too much of an advantage at this point so Pin Head started eating transdimensional meat, which he liked. It was cut from my own legs.

I planned a Christmas party as I had done on and off for years. It was to be held at Thornfield Court for the night of December 18th. I started making invitations and hired fifty pounds worth of disco lights. At the Hearing Voices Group the night before, I was a little concerned insufficient people would show up, but also a little excited. Due to the enemy, beer and wine made me feel like shit and yet sobriety seemed like a boring idea, particularly at my own party. Lacking any inspiring conversation at the Group I figured out that I could smoke hashish instead of drinking.

With enough cash in my pocket for an 8th of an ounce I told my friends I wouldn't be long and left them. I went into the night, walked into town experiencing that old familiar anxiety about 'scoring'. I needn't have worried. I went into a pub on Trinity Street and soon bought a small lump of the drug in its

303

brown resin form. I had originally planned to return triumphant but the dealer wanted to share a smoke with me. He was about five years younger and not the kind of person I would choose as a friend, but I was curious. I consented. We walked into what looked like an abandoned garage, near the St. Mary's Arts Centre, and the dealer rolled a joint. We passed it about, yet I clearly remember I had four puffs only. Four. Then I started walking back to Oxford Road feeling slightly ill like there was dry sand clogging my brain. The voices might have been quiet.

It was December 17th, eleven years to the day since I had been kicked out of college in Bristol. Back at the group I felt I ought to give a Christmas speech and I admitted I was little 'stoned', but not out of order. Then, I heard the accentless voice of someone overhead that I knew was a Cusper. He declared I had been demoted from Air-gate sergeant to Private and I felt a spore assault begin. It was very heavy. I went outside... then went back indoors. The spore in the hospital had been easier to cope with in the company of others. Not this time.

I was informed I had lost and was going to die of a blown up head. I was told to leave the building. The swell of pressure ballooning inside my skull was terrifying. I was the victim of a myth that the first man between Barker and I to use a criminal drug would lose. The war was over. In a whirlpool of dread and injustice I fell to my knees at the Group, clutching my head, and screamed. My companions couldn't have helped me even if they knew how. They may as well have been several *miles* away. The enemy wanted me to deal with it alone, to go outside and die. I kept hesitating...then I managed to say goodbye to my friends and I left the building.

On the pavement the crisis was far worse than being shot by the redundant *Triax Loritzer* – even with every pellet in the Cusper's armoury in my head at once. I could hear the chanting of alien voices that I thought were waiting Barvor, then I felt that the noise was coming from within, the noise of the spore itself. I was told to stop walking, to relax my head and let it happen. I kept walking. They said my attempts to avoid dying were pitiful and pathetic. No one cared. There may have been talk about 'swapping' after the chain of death that was to begin with me and apparently it was *my fault!!* Near the traffic lights Touleal came to say goodbye to me with an essence of knowledge that was deep and tiring. She said she was sorry about the way things had turned out; maybe we "could be together next time." This was perhaps the worst of the night but I had a destination now. I realised was walking towards the café.

Stepping into Vagabonds' warm smells of tobacco smoke and fresh coffee I brushed between the tables of a few customers to speak to a spore-controller in the restroom mirror. The tiny robot might have remembered the spore's promise to never again kill an Earth person. Hope glimmered in the glass. Whether or not it remembered that, whether or not we had been in *genuine danger*, the spore began to vent porously and a few minutes later the young man who ran the Hearing Voices Group came in. We sat together. We talked and drank tea and smoked. Marcus had a fair grasp of psychiatry. Although I may not have realised he was counselling me, he treated me as a friend. In the cab 'home' to the flat I was feeling much relief. My head felt comfortable as I sank into my bed. If I experienced any nightmares that night they could not possibly have been as traumatic as being abandoned to that terrible death. Nothing that bad would happen again.

The following night was the party. During the afternoon I cleaned, set up the disco lights, and stowed the drinks. We met at The Bell pub down the road. A few people came back to the flat, enough to make an atmosphere and I played relaxing 'house' music. It may sound amazing and enigmatic but I actually smoked dope *again* that second night! Talking in the bathroom mirror to Touleal she told me to lay off the stuff for a while and have just one more puff in about an hour and a half. I did. Watching me inhaling it the Cuspers had probably glanced at each other with a sense of amused incredulity! I had three or four puffs only and my brain ached like a sulphurous toadstool. When the last guest had left I most likely brewed tea – a nice cup of normal tea – and that would have "hit the spot". Soon I felt well enough to get into bed.

I went back to Mersea for Christmas, always a special time of year for our family. We decorated the tree, put fairy lights up around the house that looked pretty; and shiny tinsel and sprigs of holly around the pictures. Nights were warmed by a log fire in the lounge grate and sometimes I sat with a mug of tea and a fruit mince pie staring into the crackling flames. Sitting in there felt like resting your head on a warm puppy. I've never woken beside a beloved girlfriend at Christmas before but at my parents' an essence of my childhood still survived in the colourfully wrapped presents, and I liked the happy excitement.

Whatever the monsters had planned, the festivities could not be as annihilated as they had been in '97. As usual they interrupted my bedtime routine; deployed heart-box attacks and the pain of 'spike flowers' to keep me awake as long as possible. They simulated bronchitis, used a tickle between the top of my lungs and the root of my wind-pipe. The *muathryl* was cloned into seven "Moochar Attack Systems" and other strategies were planned in out-of-time-holes.

When my head was on the pillow the Boo Gimps in Gehenna repeatedly sang a French folk song for what seemed like hours, conducted by The Thrall on an inter-lace directly into my head!

Coffee did not keep me awake. It gave so much pleasure to an attending spirit I was assisted into sleep. A Bark rapturer called 'Toulon' was sure enough a fearsome sight coming down the swirling blue time tunnel into the 1.2 Line, and someone who claimed to be a 'God Of Memory Return', named Jano, came up behind me to recreate night attacks, inflict such pain. Jano was one of those monsters that didn't want to kill me, he just wanted to torture me. So I ripped his eyes out and told him that his kind of attack had no God.

The Boyes flapping around the place seemed to have become kind in their old age. As I had done with the Nullies, before, I re-named them to give them a sense of self:
"Monday Boye", "Hawk-wind Boye", "Pie Boye", and that last one loved the happy holiday so much I decided to change his name to "Christmas Boye". He put up decorations in his house hole. I wanted his Time Line to be rigged so it could be Christmas for him everyday. Exposed to loveliness like that, after so much horror, I was often torn in different emotional directions by the inevitable legacy of psychological damage.

The simulations during nights at my parents were a continuous mess. I beat the Gehennan's folk music by imagining myself breathing through my upper nose, which bypassed their inter-lace. The conductor put down his baton. I discovered that I had been the elder brother of a high God, in *physical genealogy*, and that His name was Lord God Julian. He showed me an ancient family picture of Himself as a little boy and I cried. One of the worst things the enemy did then was try to kill Him. Visual registry included images filmed on White Art cameras that were used to induce Memory Return attempts: locking images of Lord God Julian's comings and goings and perhaps attack. The badness and madness! The micro-cosmic presumptuousness and cheek of those idiot horrors! Before He left me Lord God Julian might have said *"You'll be happier than ever soon"* and it took many months to happen, years actually, but it did transpire. These days…I'm happy nearly all the time!

By Christmas Eve my gifts were wrapped. On the morrow I would give a mind speech to telepath celebrities at 11am. In my hand-written version of *"Defender"* I wrote: "I was bone tired of the conflict, by then; deep down, with no initiative, spiritually exhausted." The house that night was as warm and peaceful as a mouse. I slept well and awoke with paper crackling at the bottom of my bed. I opened the presents then went to visit the others. At eleven I sat before the mirror in the purple room and made a speech to 'subtle bodies' in an array of seats like an arena: some details are included, most are not, but here is a little more information.

Swapping their physical existences post-apocalypse, *after* an Earth 'policy', may have been a reward. Some celebrities represented Asgaroths and others Deyaforms, and maybe they changed these also. My information of the day was that it happened once every ten thousand years, when alien machines plowed the cities back into the continents. Since many earthquakes and over two centuries of archaeology haven't uncovered a single stone from one of our passed civilisations my estimation of the frequency of this must be wrong. If you look at it from the other end of time, that it has taken *billions of years* for the cycle to repeat itself, this also seems wrong: an impossibly long time. What about the dinosaurs? Had their destruction also been a 'policy'?

Whatever the duration, I had deduced a conclusion from my experiences: I had come to believe something terrible. The Earth and the souls of its peoples had been *farmed*. We had been killed by spore, raptured into *Tookle* 'fish' for Barvor's planets of 100% water, to eat us to avoid eating themselves, and the mulch that remained was sold off as Dimension Two for manufacturing *swits* and the material of the next *Helter Incendo*. Whether or not the real explanation is more 'biblical' than this, (baring in mind the Armageddon in the Book of Revelation is called *The Rapture*) it seems to me that the monster telepaths are the only people who really know what's going on and they've been lying for years!
I believed 'Revelation' had been written by Barker himself, long ago. But I hoped that by that Christmas the Earth's apocalypse was no longer considered unpreventable. After the myriad ways I had been killed down the Time Lines I revealed another belief during my speech. That Barker had

suffocated my *feelie soul* for a total of about one million years. I had been invited to speak (in my own defence, usually) a few times during 1997 but I couldn't 'see' and I didn't know how to control my *scu*. After getting bogged down in different kinds of worm attack 'wah', my speech ground to a halt of its own and was probably quickly forgotten. I went downstairs. It was Christmas Day and the warm smiles of my family were part of the reality I preferred.

I sometimes found the loveliness of my close relations ungraspable. I wanted Christmas to be a happy time, but I still had to fight. The following night, which the British call "Boxing Day", I became upset. I was bunked in the bedroom I had slept in at the beginning, so many of my weird memories absorbed into its yellow emery paper walls. I was sitting in there when I learned a contingent had been *reversing everything* I had been saying, probably on an inter-lace beyond the range of my hearing. They had been twisting my statements for months and it was hopeless.

I cried for simpler days; wept, perhaps, for a destroyed Christmas, and that same night my mother drove me to Lexden. A doctor on a call-out gave me Diazapam, after midnight. The next afternoon, December 27th, I was admitted into The Lakes again. I was to be treated for schizophrenia and depression and it was okay. I knew the 'set' and after all the attacks on my sleep if I was prescribed Zimmovane I was certainly going to take it!

Since 1990 I have been an in-patient at six different hospitals on nine occasions for over twenty-five months. Each 'set' has its own atmosphere: The optomistic holiday feeling of my recovery in Hayse Grove, the fun of socializing at The Lakes and the militant simulations at Wathamstow with all its victories and horrors. Is it easier to detect an ambience, or more difficult, when you are 'raw' in yourself? Can a very ill patient contribute to the assortment of interaction on a ward, or must healing first re-sensitize them to their surroundings? Depending on how lost you are, you usually *do* connect with others sharing that microcosm. Once, I sat up all night talking to a client and I went to bed at about 7am. When I got up at lunchtime I could barely recall a single thing we had said to each other!

In the heady times of "largin' it" in the '90s I had believed 1999 was the year of the Earth's Armageddon. My sister's boyfriend from those days, Paul Gronland, was admitted to the ward in January suffering from depression. I was surprised to see him. The New Year had come and gone with no champagne, no fanfare of trumpets…it just swept us by like a ghost ship in a fog bank. My uncle on my mother's side was on the ward also, fighting alcoholism, and he would have sorely missed that celebration, more so for being a Scott. Not just because of the myth that the Scottish drink more but because New Year is particularly important to them. January 1st clicked into place. Billions of time pieces changed and the last page of the year passed was ripped out of calendars; but I don't think any of us hardly even noticed it.

The blood-locks were still driving me to distraction. My body was shouting silently for sustenance so I had to get creative, such as chewing a little rolling tobacco whilst sipping tea. The enemy would have loved it if I chewed tobacco all the time instead of smoke. Not from any concern about my health, but because within a month my teeth would have looked like grave stones in a swamp. Chocolate felt good at bed time but I was often worried that a heart-box attack might override the maximum 15mg dose of Zimmovane. I went to sleep on my front, to present an 'upside down' perspective to an interfering enemy.

For Christmas, I had given my Dad a plinth with a bright light in it under a revolving filter. It had many changing hues shining through a sculpture of dolphins. I took it back and put a crystal tortoise on it. At night the ceiling of my room in the hospital was faceted with altering colours, a shattering of pretty revolving lights. Through the tortoise I prayed to a force that I called Lady Nature – sometimes for sleep but more regularly to be a non-telepath. I believed that She had chosen to be 'represented' by her favourite portion of mint chocolate. I ate many bars of Aero at bedtime for that dark minty smoothness in the blood. I was assaulted with spore during the days. The bladder raptures were as degrading as though I was being treated like an animal. A solid lump used to appear that felt unleakable except in a shower or (unfortunately) in a sink, while an enemy said: *"Piss like a man does!"* Yet in my mind I was getting younger.

After you've been an in-patient for six weeks your benefit money <u>was</u> drastically reduced. I had been in The Lakes for nearly five weeks. I had got what I wanted and I was thinking about going back to the flat. I had secured the vital Zimmovane prescription (with some Stelazine and Meloryl anti-psychotics as part of the package, if I wanted them) and I was still receiving Modecate 'depo' injections that I had been taking for years because they didn't do anything. The only reason I had to put up with that slightly degrading palaver was to encourage a more 'realistic' claim to sickness benefit. Yet it is a fact that while I was taking it I stayed *out of hospital* for over five and a half years. I moved back to Thornfield Court in February. The staff had suggested initially that I move into sheltered accommodation but the freedom of the flat was *my place*. I was always in the company of monsters, there, but who else could understand me? I hadn't enjoyed a long silence with my eyes open for two years.

When I was 'at home', again, I started watching TV. I saw more childrens' shows and I seemed to be regressing into a juvenile. Sometimes I held my fluffy white dog toy while my real dog Lotti was being looked after by my parents. Wet weather and an out of date tax disc scared me off riding my Honda. I often walked down the road to buy groceries. The keeper of that little shop was the *same man* that had sold me the Christmas feast in 1997, a year I reflected upon with the fondness of self-created legend. I visited his shop regularly and seeing him felt strange because he could not have known what I had gone through. I rode busses into central town to purchase toiletries, or visit the café, but I never gambled. My friends must have known I was ill but they seemed pleased to see me. In a Boots pharmacy I noticed the store's own brand of soluble Aspirin. It is a simplistic pain killer that can be dissolved in water and had always tasted foul to me but it did dull the pain sufficiently to make reaching sleep easier. Whether Aspirin was illegal or prescribed was asked repeatedly and my answer was neither. You can buy it straight off the shelf and even children can take it.

Many entities didn't treat me with a splinter of respect. The Cuspers held me in higher regard even if most of the time I didn't know if they were friend or foe. I used to salute them in mirrors. Part of me knew I might be role-playing but I wanted to be a boy. I was getting younger. I was 'going soft' more, a defence mechanism, and Lord Jon Pertwee had predicted that the war would be won by a nine year-old boy. Sometimes, in the shower and desperate to piss, Barker's own prophecy, apparently also made long ago, forecast that I would slash open my bladder with a knife. Needless to say no matter how difficult it got that horror never even came close to happening. But I needed care so I returned to Mersea, for a while.

At my parents' I discovered Belvue, a hospital Hell. It was populated by the evil mad who were 'treated' with *ratnika* and unnecessary surgery. The doctor there (soul of actor

312

Ken Granham) was hopelessly insane. In one of those rare moments of achievement there was peace between the Earth, Heaven and Hell while I was getting out of a shower. A lot of patients from Belvue were freed to migrate up to the next plane, many carrying grubby dolls with them. Barker cancelled it with memory return.

At their house I had been searching on and off for ages for a packet of Lambert & Butler cigarettes and probably decided I would find them 'when I was supposed to'. On choosing a glass from the kitchen cupboard Lady Nature may have prognosticated which glass I would choose. The first one I picked up was dirty then I pulled out a slim glass decorated with dogs. This was met with gasps of surprise so I guess it fitted the description of the glass of which Lady Nature had foretold. Sitting in the kitchen, with whatever drink I chose to put in it, a voice said: "I'll prove it to you," then told me to *look left*. I looked left and my eyes instantaneously met the packet of Lambert & Butler that was lying at the far end of the table! During the final conflict, prognostication may have been deployed by both sides. Hundreds of times the enemy have accompanied a spore assault with a count-down, but I have no essences of any real prophesy. Most of what there was had been crap and rubbish. Logically, they induced fear and may have used the like of pushed-sub-thoughts to actualise any prophesy they did do, but *very rarely*. The enemy's chosen stance was the undoing of prediction. *"Porous venting the prophesy"* they used to say. My knowledge is sketchy because I couldn't hear them being laid or else they would not have been prophesy, but the answering forces of goodness may have exercised a genuine ability to prove they had an unbeatable control over my situation.

I was trying to restrain my responses to the enemy from my parents. It was no surprise that they were unable to offer the succour I needed. My mother, particularly, seemed able to recognize when I was mentally ill: looking into my eyes, where she may have seen madness and pain, and I had to get back to the flat, back to boxing my shadow in the gladiatorial coliseum. Maybe I was escaping, running from Thornfield Court and back again. Running away from my folks and 'going soft' like an ostrich with its bum in the air that never sees the bullet coming. I was as tired as a child bullied at school day after day after day. But I went back, returned to 'Fred', and the heater, and my soft white 'cuddle dog'. It was *my* place.

I was worried about the failure of benevolent forecasting. For example, if they prophesied what time I would fall asleep I didn't want them to fail. I continued to be afraid of heart-box trouble, at bedtime, but the foul alkaline taste of soluble Aspirin helped a lot. The daily fight continued. It is difficult to say how much of what was going on I could grasp so the vave-simulation may have been adapted for a less mature outlook, but with these sadists it could have been harder than ever. The old Ellisons in Stargore put their knives down. Some had agreed weeks ago to be re-incarnated as harmless animals like squirrels and butt-eating rats. I was told of others in the place, innocents: two telepath musicians who had been friends of mine long ago. A man and a woman named (something like) John and Kathy, who had been killed at the end of the last policy, and then raptured into worm 'botnes' that were stored in a drawer in Stargore and perhaps forgotten for an age.

The harbinger of the ending of that policy began with two nuclear devices detonating in Afghanistan, a large one and a small one. On the same day, John and Kathy had been shot by Barker's hit men while performing at the Arts Centre. In the Thornfield Court (of then) I opened a bottle of red wine and I started insulting God while I was getting drunk. I had given up. I swore at Him for hours then went downstairs, lurching across the 'Y' floor, and stole a car. It was a Mini. I drove it into the pouring rain and after a complex coded number flashed before me, it was over. I never got out from behind the wheel: my head went and that's how the last policy ended. So I was told. Ever since Kathy and John had lived in that dusty drawer, in brick-down 'botnes' that had interiors like cotton wool. The couple were released and went to heaven. I don't remember hearing from Stargore again and you might agree that that is no loss.

The end of February was coming, and my victimisation may have been streamlined. The psychosis was shedding its skins like a boa constrictor. The Lord Chief Cusper shared my sister's ex-boyfriend's name. It was suggested that he was a descendant of 'a' Paul Gronland from long ago. The real Paul had been discharged from The Lakes after me and I barely remember even talking to him. The Lord Chief said he wanted to adopt me and this was good. I agreed. My belief may have helped to create the Cusper Regiment in the beginning, and my adoption in 1999 probably cued the beginning of the end, for them, the longest vave-sim of the conflict.

'Going soft' was aided by feeling hot on the inside and cold on the outside…Having a cold shower off after a long soak in the bath felt pleasant. But before it was taken away the snake took me into a new hold, with the renewed threat of heart-box pains compounded by running out of Aspirin. The following day I bought more by a different manufacturer, called *Dispirin*. I had seen them advertised on TV. I dissolved some in a glass but I measured the affective healing power of the solution by its taste and Dispirin had a sweetness like old sugar in cold tea. I either got used to it or purchased Aspirin with the taste that worked. I also took Meloryl at night with my 'sleepers' and a kind voice had said, not so long ago, that my medication would always equal sleep. I doubted that sometimes, but it did.

I went to have tea at my parents on my 30th birthday and I remember almost nothing about it. I got depressed about the tea pot and the cocktail sausages and the little sandwiches in comparison to my terrible 'life' and cried hopelessly about what little difference it made. During those cold days the worst attacks were still mostly tactile, such as the *Ratnika* spore first used when I was at school. It feels like the roots of your teeth are being electrocuted. It isn't life threatening but I felt like a whipped dog. Brushing teeth can 'vent' them, can push them away, but when re-applied they sprang back voraciously for sugars. Touleal requested *Ratnika* not be used. The enemy used it anyway, to the point of a new danger, moving beyond issues of mere cosmetics as they crept through my entire skull. Crawling, spreading, an ache designed to weaken the bone before using classic spore. Scare-mongering bullshit like: "God is now Satan" I rejected as untenable.

As usual it was always harder to dismiss what was physically verified. Lying in bed one evening peculiar inter-vicinity edible things, like sweets, were put into my hand. I ate some; and, incredibly, I could actually *taste* these things that didn't exist. Most likely a *fundament body* sitting in the 'Circle of Fire' ate them simultaneously and they tasted horrible: *Time Seeds*. I was spared knowing what they were made of – but learned Barker had gained time –control over my heart-box after I had eaten a certain number of the seeds that were designed to ruin its 'timing'. I accepted the fear of it, then, went to sleep. *"You'll never sleep peacefully again, as long as you exist"* the enemy has said over a hundred times.

I became upset in Vagabonds one afternoon. It wasn't because of my friends, my temper was frayed for telepathic reasons. I lost control and went blustering up St. John's Street where I got slightly freaked out by a toilet in a bathroom showroom. A part of me you might call "the sceptical soldier" observed the tantrum of "the abused child", with disdain. I bought a Stanley-knife from a cheap shop to 'do myself in' and I felt like I was acting, or at least as though I was attention seeking. I broke open the packet – but even if I had been *half serious* the cuts of the boy would have been rendered impossible by the man, over-ruled by bloody and unrepeatable lessons made long ago.

The Barvor attack squadrons finally arrived in April. Whales swam into my horizon, far away, and they were big inter-vicinity creatures that didn't quite exist in the Material Plane. Even without the need of armed space-ships their desires were deadly in their potential. Spore-assaulting allies and unimaginable hunger made them a mortal danger to life *and* After-Life. In West Mersea at some point, years before, I had experienced pushed-sub-thoughts that God was a whale. The *tookle* that the Barvor so craved was also inter-vicinity. I had *actually tasted* those time-seeds! I saw the whales as through a glass ceiling; bulbous, blue, hungry for our Armageddon.

I was worried about the danger to Upper Planes *feelies*, which were as harmless as Teletubbies, but they were left alone. The Barvor's jackpot was to take *all of us*, six billion people, over 50,000 times more *tookle* than available in that limited heaven. Ellison had his soul raptured into a whale.

My concentration was poor. I couldn't focus my mind on anything for long, not TV, nor a video, nor a pleasing book. One cigarette to the next kept me going, as they had always done during the worst of times. The enemy twisted the issue of temperature, reversing hot with cold saying: *"replacing blue Quiddity with black Diddity"* and I was black and blue myself, fidgeting with my duvet and turning the heater on and off in climatic confusion. Thus they took away my 'going soft', inducing secondary stress-related illnesses.

A large number of whales 'held off', in orbit, around our planet. Other's developed communication. I sent imagination-created Dimension Three attack spore right up their inter-lace lines, their robot brains crashed and their bodies fell out of the sky like air-ships. Barker may have had his soul raptured into a whale as well, one of those things that they *only wanted me to know*. Equally damning was that other whales may have had old Barker and Ellison souls from past policies. The battles raged, spore flew back and forth; the situation was not actually 'going anywhere' until a whale squadron leader introduced himself as *Meloryl*. It was the brand name of an anti-psychotic I was supposed to take. It was a curious opportunity.

I started focussing on the principal issues: a hunger so profound that if the Barvor didn't eat us they would eat themselves unto their own extinction. Something had to be done. The ultimate example of the "kick & kiss" initiative, else it would reinforce the war for the survival of one planet. The answer came from heaven. After I had learned *feelies* have magic plates and cutlery that cleaned themselves. I wondered…where did their food come from? And I found out! When they were hungry they got tasty magic dinners in little packages that appeared through White Rapture. The whales were similar to us in that they could 'brick-down' also, into their own mouths. I started to join the dots, and while staying at my parents I went for the Answer.

I went for "The Key to the City", found a practitioner of White Magic who could conjure up the magic food and encouraged him to share his 'tech' with the Barvor. Parcels appeared in the mouths of Meloryl's whales. Warm tookle-flavour rolls wrapped in colourful paper and tied up with bows! The Barvor had food, now, and they said it was delicious. I was in the yellow bedroom when Barker counter-attacked, casting a black rapture to make them feel sick. I was in dread of the Barvor thinking their suppers were to blame but they must have known. Because they may have all left our planet by the time I returned to the flat. The conjuration spread through the ranks, fast, as good news does. If they hadn't left the Earth before my return, then they did soon. Such beginnings are always delicate but they could adapt the dinners – and leave us alone. Like the Alphas' before them, attempts were made to memory return the whales but they did not want to be brought back. As I wrote in my original version: *"(they) had learnt to hate Barker's war-stirring in favour of peace meals. Thus, ended the huger issues. The Barvor did not want anyone to re-dress the conflict."*

A large part of me believed all of it, that I had become the last line of defiance and we had won. I was emotionally depleted but much of the danger to our planet went with the whales. I couldn't be bothered with Thornfield Court anymore. The Earth was safe. The globally destructive motives of my enemies had been made non-viable, yet I don't think I grasped the enormity of this victory. I remember saying our survival meant a future with 'light speed engines'. Although I wasn't going to invent this myself, such a thing is not so unlikely to come to pass. And what of the utter unimaginable horror of defeat? To the better part of me that had always been impossible!

I was a half-demolished sculpture of my former self, leaning over, and near complete collapse. Life at the flat had become unsustainable. I'm not saying I would have died if I had stayed there, because I don't think I would have done, but I had been tortured enough. There was one hope only of salvation from utter disintegration, to volunteer for mental health treatment so I packed a bag with clothes, and 'Fred', and my big cuddle-dog, and Dad dropped me off at The Lakes. It was no blemish on my accomplishments as a *Defender*. The fearful exhaustion of post traumatic stress and other derived illnesses were another, more genuine reality, sufficiently disabling for me to accept psychiatry with an open heart, maybe for the first time.

Once I was back in the hospital I was to recover – but it seemed that no one had told the enemy that the war was over. The toilet stuff remained blocked. The spore-assaults continued. The blood-locks were now strong enough to exclude even sugars. I was like the only survivor of a sunken ship that had been washed up on the bland beach of Gosfield ward, feeling stunned, wandering about aimlessly and alone except for a cuddly toy. The things that had kept me going: tea, chocolate, coffee, cigarettes: again they filled me with an over stuffed brain-taste while almost *none of it* flowed around my blood stream. The Lakes was not a 'set' this time. I felt that I was very ill.

Doctor Baloche had been my consultant in 1990 and was now again, in 1999. I told her I would do her will, take any medication she prescribed – except *Chlorpromazine* – because it was my only chance of being free of these cursed voices that I had fought for so long. She raised my 'depo' injections of *Modecate*, twice, up to 150ml every ten days but that exaggeration was apparently useless and soon cancelled. On the wards, I often had a sense of indefinable panic, like I was the only living fish left in an empty aquarium, so I was given a *Benzodiazepine* to help cope with this anxiety. Small blue 1mg granules of *Lorazapam* that the Lower Plane *feelies* and the interior *scu*, particularly liked a lot; as usual maybe too much!

I took other anti-psychotic drugs. At the beginning of my treatment, I used to employ percentage 'reaches' to estimate which tablets would be the most affective at reducing the 'voices'. At weekly reviews I told my doctor that I was on miraculous medication, like *Haloperidol*, but two weeks later I would often tell her it wasn't working. Given half a chance I had thrown out most drugs like this in the past. In fact I had never even *tried* many of them and that's why in Doctor Baloche's reality she and her colleagues had prescribed a lot of drugs that hadn't worked. Thus she chose *Clozapine*, one of the new 'A-typical' anti-psychotics. The brand name is *Clozaril* and it is like Lithium in that it is a drug that builds up in the blood, but there the similarity ends.

Clozaril has a list of potentially debilitating side-affects as long as your arm, yet it is considered the last bastion of help after all else has failed. The last hope for many "who are unresponsive or intolerant to conventional neuroleptics", so says the patient's hand book. Doctor Baloche felt it was serious enough to seek a second opinion. An appointment was made for me to go up The Maudsley Hospital, in London, and be assessed by a doctor on 10th May. It had surprised me. I had never heard of Doctor Baloche doing the like of it before.

According to a 'sliding scale' system that the staff exercised, they raised the dose of the new medication and gradually phased out <u>all the other drugs</u> on my card, except for the max 15mg dose of *Zimmovane*. *Closapine* can cause neutropenia, affecting white corpuscles, so regular blood-tests must go to the Clozaril Monitoring Service: green to continue, red to halt, and orange to re-test. It would take six months to a year to work. And that was one of the reasons I believed it might actually free me.

I used to say *Lorazapam* "crunches like Marlboro" and the interior *scu* often reduced me to a state like panic-stricken mashed potato in order to get a fix of it. The consultant assessing me in London gave *Clozaril* the rubber stamp. She also proscribed an anti-depressant, let me choose one of two, and that was lucky for me because this sliding scale meant that I was <u>affectively on nothing</u> for about six weeks. The addicted *scu* had to accept that whatever the anxiety they generated they would not be able to get *Benzodiazepines* anymore. I was having a rough time myself!

I needed to be hugged, needed to be touched. I was as harmless as a mouse in a maze oblivious to the experiment, but tactile affection from nursing staff remains prohibited. In the evenings I just wanted to sit about comfortably holding cuddle-dog, and sometimes I used to sit beside a very old lady on the sofa in the Ardleigh ward smoking lounge. Her name was Iris. After a half dose of Zimmovane I used to sit so that she could hold my left hand. She softly rubbed the terrible scars with her fingertips and I felt her love. If I was sixty 60 + years old I might have married her myself. I told her so! Usually, after the enemy had stopped blathering on about milk and cigarette use being *'an eternal fix-head',* and after a couple of grand yawns, I would take the other sleeping tablet and shuffle off to bed.

Some nights weren't quite that easy. I would hug cuddle-dog in an anxious delirium around midnight in the doorway of the Gosfield Ward Nursing Station. A locked-moment like a question mark, shifting from foot to foot saying: "I don't know what to do! *I don't know what to do!*" over and over, again. But even if the Night Staff had wanted to they couldn't help me with tablets. There were no P.R.Ns, nothing extra written on my medication card. One of the staff, Dawn, used to ask: "What would you normally do at a time like this?" and I spoke of making toast, or tea, or writing a letter to Touleal as I did most days. I usually ended up watching TV on *Zimmovane* until I was sufficiently relaxed.

I wondered if my consultant actually knew anything about my experiences. I was interviewed by her *locum* assistants, and told them some of it, wanting to open up. After my Doctor's liaisons with them I saw her at a weekly review and she told me my psychosis was like a script for a *Star Wars* film! Talking about the unbelievable isn't always a waste of breath. I started seeing a pretty patient called Rachel, who looked like a kissable newsreader. Someone put cuddle-dog in a washing-machine and I was worried but I laughed to see his face going round and round through the window. I began to get into routines. Not just for survival, but also for recovery. I asked for my hot food to be put in a bowl and took it into the garden. At twilight I sometimes ate at a table listening to the beautiful song of a black bird, perhaps the same bird that had returned to roost at the same time every night since I had last been in the hospital during February.

Rachel was also schizophrenic. She heard nasty 'voices' herself. The problem with inter-patient relationships, such as ours, is that when one person gets better faster than the other, maintaining a balance of feeling between the couple can become difficult. It did cause me anxiety but my anti-depressant seemed to be cheering me up. I visited the art room and tried to communicate more with other service users. Before bed, I sometimes sat in the freshness of the Gosfield Quiet Room on the sofa in just a dressing gown: holding cuddle-dog in the darkness listening to classical music on the radio – Classic FM or Radio Three – until yawned as widely as a French Horn… and I *did* sleep. My haematology monitoring visits were re-organised, spread more widely across each month, and I was getting better – maybe happier than I had felt for years. Time was passing and brought freedom with it.

I don't think I ever believed utterly that *Closapine* was my last hope for a life but it seemed to be taking me there anyway. Shortly before I left Gosfield Ward an 'after-care package' was put together during a C.P.A meeting, and I was discharged from The Lakes on 23rd June 1999. I have continued to take *Clozapine* at the dose originally prescribed and I have never been back to any hospital like it since.

Thornfield Court was sold (at a small profit!) and I moved into a sheltered housing project in Colchester called Ashliegh Homes. I should have moved into a place like it long, long, ago but I had been a *Defender* then. A different man. My room had possibilities; at the top, on the third floor, where I happily made friends. I painted a new series of 'Blue Vortex' pictures in the lounge. They were richer and had deeper colours than those of '97, pure water-based oil colour thickly textured with brush and fingertip. I placed the new paintings and some of my old ones around the lounge, a little like a gallery, so I thought. There was soft furniture and a TV, and massive west-facing windows, a place to cement friendships. I wasn't reading much, yet Stephen King had penned in his book *"On Writing"* that if you don't read, you can't write. I made weak attempts to start a novel from an old idea that I looked upon years later as too hurtfully 'nuclear'. I watched TV and purchased a new stereo. I enjoyed videos from my growing collection of V.H.S.

A man that I had originally met in Myland Court West, in 1990, moved from The Lakes into the project within the same fortnight I did! We shared kitchen facilities and had archetypal arguments about the mess. I stayed up all night sometimes, made dance tracks with my mate Ralph using

Music 2000 on the original PlayStation. You can never have too many good friends.

Unfortunately my kissable newsreader Rachel had also been discharged, and she had moved back to a place many miles away called Halstead. She didn't seem to like telephones and we drifted apart. I still heard my enemy 'voices' but now I had some cutting edge advantages over them: a moderated but functional *Zimmovane* prescription; *Remegel* to cure heart-box pain within a minute; and a whopping great dose of 800mg of *Closapine* per day without <u>one single noticeable</u> side-affect! The spore assaults continued for brief moments, but (as I have already written) a weapon used too much loses its effectiveness. I liked where I was living and the sun shone down, but there was the possibility of trouble ahead in the form of a full solar eclipse on 11th August. No doubt the enemy were hatching nasty plots for that one – but I had a plan of my own.

There are members of staff on duty here at Ashleigh Homes 'twenty-four-seven' but it isn't a hospital. We have our own keys and can come and go as we please. One can enjoy solitude here just as easily as seek a confidant. Sheltered housing has been good for me, so I have repeatedly told people recovering from mental illness that are excited about moving into their own flats that loneliness can be dangerous... Seal's head, rotating on a green background and sparkling with bolts of electricity, singing: *"It's the loneliness that's the Killer."* The full solar eclipse on the 11th would have inspired much dread in pre-*Closapine* days, but I countered whatever simulation the enemy had planned *by being asleep*. I woke up afterwards all the happier for having missed it! Summer days drifted into winter darkness with calendar pages falling like leaves.

If someone asks my opinion about population growth, I might like to answer, if I can remember to say it: "The more the merrier!" In 1900, pundits had forecast that by 1950 we'd be knee deep in horse-shit but we invented the internal-combustion engine. If asked my views on the ceaseless number of vehicles clogging the roads now, more with every sunrise, I would answer that Mankind can be very inventive when our collective back is against the wall and we'll invent flying cars. Because we are an adaptable race, or else we might as well throw in the towel and let Cronenberg study it in an out-of-time-hole. Here's a tricky hypothesis I will call 'The Reality Question': If you believe every challenge I faced had been simulated did I ever *actually save* anyone? Since others believed that the world may not have survived if I died – so, being subjected to simulations engineered to wear me down, and kill me – when I beat *those* I saved not only myself, but may have also saved the world as a consequence! Bring forth the hand-basket!!

I returned to the flat at Thornfield Court later, to take B&W photographs. The 'Y' floor seemed to have retained the intensity of a near-death experience. The balcony rail and the wooden steps leading up to it still looked like a scaffold. I wondered who was living up there now and if there was a bad atmosphere like my experiences had soaked into the walls to cause ghostly visions that walked in daylight and bad dreams. I was torn between wanting to leave it or live in it, like Stockholm Syndrome – the relationship between kidnapper and captive – just a quick look... please... *just for a moment*...

I enjoyed staying at my parents at Christmas. My mother said 1999 was one of the best celebrations our family had shared for years. I came off my anti-depressants accidentally, didn't take them for a few days and slid from that slightly 'smoky' well being into a bigger personal reality as our race moved towards a new millennium. I felt a clarity that glittered. I skipped out of a party on the 31st and was on the top floor of Ashleigh Homes where I watched New Year's Eve celebrations take place on television. Saw the endeavour of the BBC broadcasting from far away places in different time-zones, each country joyfully celebrating as the clock ticked inexorably towards Greenwich and toward us, like the approach of a delightful and glorious bird.

I was facing west at the windows when our midnight came. After a count-down by crowds of revellers the Year 2000 was marked with tonnes of fire-works painting colourful explosions over the River Thames. At the same moment I watched the horizon over the town I so loved, Colchester, from three stories up also sparkling with glittering and crackles and sky-bursts like flowers. I wept with joy.

The fire-works I was seeing were very different from the fire that could have been. The nuclear fire I had expected as a younger and perhaps darker man had not taken a single life. The Earth still turned, and our people were alive. There was gigantic party going on and I was leaving behind a lot of horror with along the 20th century. Gone into history were two physical World Wars and the idea that the 3rd World War had been fought in the mind, and that the worst of it had been won by the side of Good. The enemy won't admit that just yet, but they will. And when they do I won't be able to hear them.

THE END